*Praise for*

# GOLD MEDAL SLEEP

"*Gold Medal Sleep* deserves a place among the classics of modern sleep writing. Brad Wolgast speaks directly to readers with warmth, clarity, and a rare kind of honesty that instantly builds trust. Too many insomnia self-help books rely on fear and intimidation to drive change; this one takes the more effective and humane path of growth through education. It's funny when it needs to be, scientifically rigorous throughout, and consistently engaging. Humans may indeed be the only animals capable of developing a sleep disorder simply by worrying about sleep, but we are also the only ones clever enough to write books like this that fix it."

**W. CHRIS WINTER**, MD, author of *The Sleep Solution* and *The Rested Child*

"In *Gold Medal Sleep*, Dr. Brad Wolgast provides a brief, accessible, and friendly introduction to the science of behavioral sleep and circadian health. It is practical, straightforward, and easy to read, but it also keeps itself firmly planted in established, well-validated sleep strategies. Rather than chasing trends, Dr. Wolgast reminds readers of the power of the fundamentals and maintaining a healthy frame of reference when approaching sleep health."

**MICHAEL GRANDNER**, PhD, MTR, CBSM, FAASM, director of the Sleep and Health Research Program, University of Arizona, and director of the Behavioral Sleep Medicine Clinic, Banner-University Medical Center

"Dr. Wolgast brings together his personal experiences and professional expertise to offer a compelling and accessible approach to resetting the circadian rhythm through the idea of 'camping in.' The idea is simple, elegant, and aligns beautifully with what we know about sleep science. This is a warm, engaging, and practical guide that reflects Dr. Wolgast's clinical skill and his genuine care for the people he serves."

**KRISTI E. PRUIKSMA**, PhD, DBSM, professor, Department of Psychiatry and Behavioral Sciences, University of Texas Health at San Antonio

BRAD WOLGAST
PhD, DBSM

# GOLD MEDAL SLEEP

## THE EVERYPERSON'S GUIDE for Restful Nights, Energetic Days, and a Healthy Life

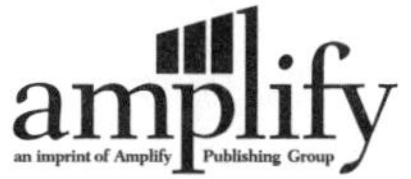

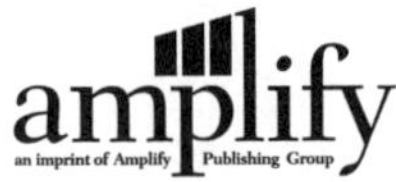

www.amplifypublishinggroup.com

*Gold Medal Sleep: The Everyperson's Guide for Restful Nights, Energetic Days, and a Healthy Life*



**For more information, please contact:**
Amplify Publishing, an imprint of Amplify Publishing Group
620 Herndon Parkway, Suite 220
Herndon, VA 20170
info@amplifypublishing.com

Library of Congress Control Number: 2025927131

CPSIA Code: PRV0126A

ISBN-13: 979-8-89138-964-9

Printed in the United States

*For Lisa—for everything.*

# CONTENTS

# PROLOGUE

As a sleep professional, one of my most rewarding activities is giving talks to practitioners and the public about sleep. Unfortunately, there is precious little education about sleep provided to students and the public these days that is reliable and not tied to some sort of product or medication to buy.

Don't get me wrong; there are outstanding resources for reliable, science-based sleep information out there, including great books, podcasts, and websites (some of which I will reference at the end of this book). Unfortunately, most of what people hear about sleep is from an advertisement for a new sleep medication.

In my practice as a sleep psychologist, the most common question I receive from clients and in presentations is, "What tips can help me sleep better?" A colleague of mine and I joke about paying each other a dollar every time we go over these same suggestions. The same dollar would go back and forth between our offices, sometimes several times a day, and would never get spent.

And another question we hear repeatedly is, "How do I get the best night of sleep every night?" No one has perfect sleep because we are humans, not machines, and you can't expect to have the best sleep every night. Even great sleepers have bad nights from time to time. But can you improve your daily routines to make good, consistent sleep more likely? Absolutely.

This book will walk you through the realities of modern living that make sleep challenging, from your phone to your kitchen lights. I will explain how things got this way and why it is so challenging for so many people to sleep well these days. Then, I will provide you with my top suggestions for better sleep and how to circumvent the disruptions to your body's natural ability to promote sleep. Because no two of us are alike and because your motivations to sleep are different from the next person reading this book, I will guide you through three levels of improvement for your sleep goals: bronze, silver, and gold. There aren't any medals for achieving these levels, and the gold level may not be for you, or not for you all the time. That's okay! My goal is to provide you with ideas, direction, and an understanding of why you should select new routines and improve your old routines for sleep in a way that fits your lifestyle.

And finally, I'll put all these tips and ideas together for you in a package I call the *Camping Sleep Reset*. If you don't like camping, don't worry! You won't have to leave home to do it.

This book will provide you with several techniques that just about anyone can use starting today. There are reasons that these steps may not work for you (especially for those of you who are shift workers or who have addiction issues). If you need more help, reach out to your primary care doctor or a local sleep expert. To help you find one, try the SBSM website: https://www.behavioralsleep.org/index.php/united-states-sbsm-members

Good luck with your sleep journey. Remember that your sleep will happen even if you get in the way.

—BW, 2025

INTRODUCTION

# WHY AM I HERE?

I'm passionate about sleep. I have been my whole life. I learned very early on that I could never have too much sleep. As a kid, my parents were caring, thoughtful, and respectful of the medical world: If a medical doctor told them what to do, it was trusted as truth. It's a safe bet to trust people who spend years learning medical science to provide you with solid advice and care—it's what I do today. However, in the 1970s physicians weren't trained to look for potential problems with sleep, especially with children. As a result, even though I snored loudly enough to be heard in another room, neither my parents, my pediatrician, nor anyone else ever considered that my snoring might be a reason for medical concern.

As I got older, my brother nicknamed me "Chainsaw Brad" because sleeping in the same room with me was a little bit like sleeping in the same room with a chainsaw. I would snore throughout the night consistently, and I was loud. By the time I was a young teenager, I would often wake up with a headache and dry mouth. My tongue would be dried out because I slept with my mouth open all night. In fact, I could only breathe if my mouth was open. I never wondered if it wasn't healthy because this was literally the only way I had ever breathed.

As kids in the 1970s, my brother and I would watch TV after school. Some of our favorite things to watch were what we would call "cops and robbers" shows. You know, where a "bad guy" does something and the police work to catch him. (This was a long time before *CSI*.) I remember the first time I watched a kidnapping where the bad guy took the hero as a hostage and then taped his mouth shut to keep him from yelling. When I saw this, I said, "Oh no! He'll suffocate!" My brother laughed at me and said, "What are you talking about?" as a good older brother would and then looked at me like I was crazy. It was clear that I had a fundamental misunderstanding of how breathing worked. I didn't understand it at the time, but I did know that if I kept my mouth closed for too long, or if someone taped my mouth shut, I would probably pass out from lack of oxygen. Mental note to myself as a seven-year-old: *Do not get taken hostage.*

During my school years, I used to catch every virus and infection that came through school. I was sick during school breaks and when school was in session, and I would spend weekends catching up on sleep or getting rid of a cold. I had enough ear infections to get tubes and enough strep throat that I knew the names of the antibiotics that were available about as well as my pediatrician. My friends used to joke that the school nurse should have a meeting with me every Monday morning to find out what I had been fighting off so that she would know what to look for.

I had difficulty staying awake every day during high school. While I was an active and successful high school student, I struggled with driving a car. It was a challenge for me to stay awake during the entire red light waiting for the green. I drove around with a six-pack of Jolt

Cola ("All the sugar! Twice the Caffeine!") in the back of my Toyota until one hot day when the four remaining cans exploded. I had difficulty studying in the evenings after school because I would simply fall asleep. I struggled with sitting down to read because I would fall asleep within a few minutes. Sitting in class, I could stay awake, but it was a struggle. I learned tricks to prevent nodding off that were sometimes effective. When I was in high school in the 1980s, unlike today, drinking coffee was something for old people. For me to drink coffee in high school would have felt as normal as dressing up like my grandfather. So coffee was not something I used to stay awake.

As luck would have it, when I was in my senior year of high school and playing basketball, I was hit in the jaw and knocked to the court. While I felt okay, I wound up in the examination room with an outstanding ear nose and throat doctor, Dr. Song Ping Lee. Dr. Lee examined me and was quick to say, "Your jaw is fine; I'm not worried about that. But how do you breathe through your nose?"

I will never forget looking at him and saying, "I never have."

Dr. Lee said, "Let's fix this."

That day, my life changed.

I learned that day that I was born with a significantly deviated septum. Many people have a mildly or moderately deviated septum. Some are born with it, like me; others have a deviated septum caused by bike accidents, fights, or falls. Throughout my early life, this septum prevented me from being able to breathe through my nose, and at night, it created septum-based obstructive sleep apnea. A few months after meeting with him, Dr. Lee operated on my nose to fix the deviated septum and sent me home to recover and start my new life.

Over the next several months, as my nose and nasal passages healed, I began to experience for the first time in my life what it was like to have restful, healthy sleep and to live with consistent energy. My life changed completely.

I could now confidently stay awake in my car during an entire red light. I was able to study. I was able to read for longer than fifteen minutes at a time. In fact, I could read for long periods of time, like everyone else! All of this was possible because I was finally able to sleep effectively. I could spend time with friends later into the evening. I could enjoy being with people and doing things I enjoyed without worrying how long I'd be able to stay awake. I was funnier. I was kinder. I was more curious. I was less irritable. It was an amazing transformation for me.

This led to a profound appreciation for and enjoyment of healthy sleep. Not only was I thrilled to have energy and thoughtfulness, but also, I was healthier. I wasn't catching colds, getting sick, and having headaches, a dry tongue, and jaw aches. In addition, my mental health improved; I wasn't frustrated by chronic fatigue and its constant wear and tear on me. I was neither exhausted all the time nor easily irritated by my friends and family members. I was able to relax more easily and enjoy myself more thoroughly. I even found and took a psychology class called "Sleep and Dreaming" with Dr. Charles Hallenbeck at the University of Kansas—one of the first of its kind. I fell in love with the science of sleep.

After I recovered and had a successful freshman year in college, I decided it was time to maximize my health and do something I loved during my summers. I worked as a backpacking guide in the largest private wilderness camping area in the world—Philmont Scout Ranch, in the mountains of New Mexico. Here, over 140,000 acres, I honed my outdoor skills, spending very few hours under a roof and nearly all my time outdoors and sleeping outside every night all summer. These were days of exertion: lots of hiking, lots of sweating, and lots of training young campers how to carry a thirty-pound backpack for hours each day and enjoy the experience. Those days and nights became inspiration for this book. You'll hear about how camping (outside AND inside!) promotes sleep and how you can use the vital aspects of *Camping In* in your daily life to obtain similar gains.

After college, it was clear to me that I wanted to be a psychologist because I wanted to help people deal with some of the most difficult times and mental health experiences of their lives. I went to Philadelphia for my graduate work at Temple University. I didn't know it at the time, but Philadelphia was on its way to becoming a sleep medicine and behavioral sleep medicine epicenter. I sought a doctorate in psychology, and when kids would ask me what my job was, I'd tell them I was still in school—in the twenty-second grade.

Eventually, my job was being a therapist. I was most likely drawn to therapy with university students at counseling centers because my most challenging and formative years happened in college. I started college as a young man with a sleep disorder who fell asleep reading more than a few pages. I finished college with my health, my sleep, and my life in order.

It was the students I met with and provided therapy to during my nine years at the University of Pennsylvania's counseling center who inspired me to dig deeper into sleep. They were experiencing anxiety, depression, eating disorders, thoughts of suicide, panic, heavy drug use, mania, and even psychosis. But there was an underlying theme across all my clients—they weren't sleeping well.

The University of Pennsylvania and the Children's Hospital of Philadelphia next door happen to have some of the most respected behavior sleep medicine researchers and clinicians in the world. I was introduced to Phil Gehrman, PhD, and Jodi Mindell, PhD, and both were excited by my interest in sleep. These two are important researchers in the field of sleep, and they welcomed me into their discussion and were just as excited about sleep as I was, which was new to me. They suggested readings; they told me about conferences; they helped me see the possibilities for more training and eventually certification.

Phil agreed to oversee my efforts as I worked on my board certification for behavior sleep medicine. Over the course of about eighteen months, I studied, I saw more clients struggling with sleep than ever, and Phil supervised my clinical care. Then I took one of the most difficult exams I've ever taken—the behavioral sleep medicine certification exam. This is what it means to be board certified. A board of professionals in behavior sleep medicine creates these training requirements and a three-hour exam. Those who complete the requirements and pass the exam can say that they are board certified in behavior sleep medicine. And in 2012, the American Board of Sleep Medicine made me the 382nd person in the world to do so. Yes, there are more letters after my name, but more than that—when you see CBSM or DBSM after a name, it means that person is more experienced and trained than the rest of the field.

These days, I manage my own private sleep practice. I work with people who have chronic insomnia (the average time my clients suffer from insomnia before I meet with them: fifteen years) or chronic nightmares. I consult with business leaders, high-level athletes, human resources departments, universities, colleges, and school boards about their concerns about sleep. I also am a member of the accreditation committee for the Society for Behavioral Sleep Medicine because I believe it is vital for mental health providers to have opportunities that provide excellent training in sleep as well as prepare them for board certification. We need more people who do this!

I wrote this book because I believe that sleep is your superpower. I found that out when I went from sleeping terribly to sleeping very well over the course of a few months in college. (Thanks, Dr. Lee!) I have learned how powerful sleep is in improving mental health, physical health (think: heart disease, dementia, and diabetes), and inoculation health (think: the flu). The benefits of sleep include injury prevention and recovery, increased athletic ability, and better memory, creativity, friendliness, kindness, warmth, and tolerance. I think all of us would welcome these elements in bigger doses in our lives.

Whether you are looking to improve your own sleep or are a mental health provider, physician, PA, physical therapist, nurse, or someone else in a health-related field, I hope you'll use what you learn here to boost both your own sleep and the sleep of those you serve. You'll be presented with information about why sleep is vital and how many of us interfere with this critical drive. I will teach you about your sleep and present strategies on how to improve it on a day-to-day level.

I have worked with young adults and college students for the last twenty-five years. My professional area of expertise since before the millennium has been college students and their experience with mental health and sleep problems. During that time, I have also trained hundreds of psychologists, psychiatrists, psychiatric nurse practitioners, social workers, mental health workers, and other health care practitioners about the basics of sleep, including how to recognize and treat sleep problems and how to encourage healthier sleeping behaviors for better living.

This book is for everyone—the occasional poor sleeper, the health care professional looking to improve their work, and the people out there who are dealing with something more significant in their sleep life. I want to help you learn how to improve your sleep abilities. Thanks for being here. Thank you for your interest in sleep. Good luck with your sleep journey.

**Brad Wolgast, PhD, DBSM**

*All of humanity's problems stem from man's inability to sit quietly in a room alone.*

**—Blaise Pascal, *Pensées***

*Over recent decades we have come from dwelling in an outer world in which the living works of nature either predominated or were near at hand, to dwelling in an environment dominated by a technology which is wondrously powerful and yet nonetheless dead, inanimate.*

**—Harold Searles, 1960**

CHAPTER 1

# WHAT'S THE PROBLEM HERE?

It's Tuesday. It's 7:25 a.m. The alarm is going off for the third time, and you are looking at it with one eye open, trying to remember if it's Friday or Saturday. You are thinking that another two hours of sleep would probably be enough, but you must be at work, and that's not going to happen. You drag yourself out of bed and get your morning started. It is slow; it is unpleasant; it is nothing that the coffee or toothpaste commercials promise your mornings will be. And it feels like this nearly every day.

At work, people around you complain that they feel tired all the time. Some of them have problems sleeping; some have very young kids who keep them awake; some have partners (or dogs!) who snore and wake them up all night. But not you. You have a quiet enough, dark enough bedroom, there are no competing demands for your attention, and you are pretty darn healthy. Does this sound familiar? Why is it that you spend most of your weeks wishing you could lie down or just sleep a little longer?

That was how life was for Alex before she and I worked on her sleep, and she "camped in" to reset her sleep. Like all the people I reference in this book, Alex is a combination of clients whom I've worked with. I've woven together my work with them into client stories.

These days, Alex wakes up in the morning sometimes with her alarm, sometimes without it. She feels pretty alert when she wakes up. It still isn't as good as the toothpaste commercials show you, but it's better than what you have been feeling. She has some breakfast while reading the news, gets dressed, and goes to school—she is a first-year medical student. When you learn that her first cup of coffee each day is between 9:00 a.m. and 10:00 a.m., you wonder how she makes it so long. You also know that she finishes drinking coffee just after lunch but still seems alert and engaged throughout the afternoon. And you know she has been training for a 10K running race after classes with a friend.

What is going on here? Why is Alex so different from you?

What if I told you that two years ago, Alex's mornings were just like yours? What if I told you that after she went to her doctor and got blood tests to rule out medical causes for her groggy life, she began meeting with me and changed her lifestyle in ways that were mostly free but required a few personal sacrifices? She didn't change her diet. She didn't add supplements. She didn't pay for a subscription to a service that would monitor her health data. She changed how she approached her day: how she prepared for sleep, how she woke up from sleep, and, once or twice a week, she acted like the power was out when she gets home from medical school.

As a result, Alex now goes to sleep a bit earlier (because she is feeling sleepy), gets a bit more sleep, craves cookies and sweets far less than she used to, and describes herself feeling calmer, less moody, and more engaged in her life. When she and I met for the first time, she was frustrated, irritable, sleepy, and feeling doomed in both academics and her relationship. Now she has a new relationship with school and studying, is preparing to get engaged because she has gotten closer to her girlfriend, and talks about how relaxed she feels—not tired. She says the quality of her life has improved "one hundred percent."

My clients come to me for many sleep-related reasons. Before I began specializing in sleep, I was a general practitioner. While the number one complaint from clients has varied between depression and anxiety, the second complaint is usually fatigue, exhaustion, tiredness, or low energy. In addition, once I learned that the first symptom of an overall reduction in sleep is irritability, I began to notice that most of the irritable clients I met were also undersleeping.

And it surprised no one when Earl Ford's 2015 research showed that the number of American adults who slept 6 hours or fewer increased 31% over a twenty-year period, or about 70 million people. Six hours of sleep may not sound like much less than eight until you consider that, compared to your grandparents, an estimated one in four US sleepers is getting 1.5 fewer nights of sleep per week. That is a lot of lost sleep. To put it another way, your grandparents probably slept an average of about 73 more nights per year than a quarter of your friends and family now do. Since irritability is the first sign of being underslept, and so many American adults sleep 73 nights fewer per year than their grandparents did, is it any wonder that people seem more edgy and less tolerant now?

I invite you to join Alex and me in changing your sleep experience. In this book I will show you the unseen but readily available path to getting more sleep, better rest, and better overall human alignment with how your body was designed to operate.

The pathway will start with an understanding of who we are as humans. This means understanding how we were designed to operate in the world for the last few million years and then understanding what is getting in our way from that now. Ready to get started?

## IT'S NOT EASY, BEING HUMAN

If you are reading this, you probably have had more than your share of nights when you wished your sleep were better. Maybe more sleepless nights than good nights. If you think you might have a sleep disorder, you should consult with your primary care physician and follow up with any referrals you are given for specialists. Millions of Americans are suffering from undiagnosed sleep disorders. Reading this book isn't going to cure disorders. This book is not medical advice, and it is not intended as treatment for any sleep disorder.

Also, you are a human being, and that comes with advantages and disadvantages. In 1990, *Time* magazine had an article titled, "Evolution, Extinction and the Movies," that quoted Stephen Jay Gould as saying, "People talk about human intelligence as the greatest adaptation in the history of the planet. It is an amazing and marvelous thing, but in evolutionary terms, it is as likely to do us in as to help us along." When I read this quote, I immediately think of sleep. Humans appear to be the only animals on the planet who can develop a sleep disorder by worrying whether we will be able to sleep. Worrying about sleep is uniquely human. This is likely due to having a much larger frontal lobe than other animals. Thanks, evolution! What that means is that our big brains helped us create air conditioning, mobile phones, *and* the ability to worry about things that aren't really problems, like being unable to sleep.

Let me back up. What many of us are unaware of is that sleep is a basic drive for living. All animals and most plants have a sleep cycle or something like it. With too little sleep, our organs start functioning more poorly, we have difficulty fighting illnesses and recovering from injury, and our mental health deteriorates. You've probably heard too much of what goes wrong with too little sleep.

Sleep is a drive. Other drives are hunger, thirst, and breathing. It's a pretty short list. Without nutrition, water, oxygen, and sleep, we will die. Ever get so thirsty that you couldn't think about anything except finding water? Ever hold your breath under water so long you started to panic? This is how your brain operates to keep you alive when your drive to survive is impeded. It is the same with sleep, only slower. Have you ever been awake so long that you began to nod off in the middle of something important? That is your sleep drive acting on you—taking advantage of your weakened state to grab some sleep, even if for just a few moments.

The truth is that because of your sleep drive, **your body will get the sleep it needs.** Under extreme stress (a car accident, dealing with divorce, being fired from a job, etc.), your mind can convince your body that it needs to be vigilant more than it needs sleep. When it does, your sleep can be overridden briefly. But not for long. You can get distressed enough to prevent sleep for a night, maybe two. If you are good at it, you can keep yourself from sleeping for three nights entirely. Beyond that, it takes a special person with highly advanced anxiety or distress to go without any sleep for more than three nights. If you are one of those people, I'm sorry. The good news here is that extreme stress is usually so distressing that the lack of sleep is the least of your concerns, and when things settle down from the stressor, the sleep happily returns.

But very few of you can do that. There are many of you right now who read the last paragraph and are saying, "Not me; I haven't slept at all in weeks/months/years." If that sounds like you, I'm going to politely disagree. I'll ask you to finish this book first, then read *The Sleep Solution* by W. Chris Winter and get back to me.

In spite of these stressful times, our bodies will sleep nightly. **Your body will get the sleep it needs.** When you experience moderate stress (e.g., an upcoming presentation, a disagreement at work, or losing your wallet) you may lose some sleep, but you will also get some sleep. These are the nights that can lead down the road to developing insomnia if you aren't careful. If you expect to sleep but cannot and then begin to worry why you can no longer sleep, you can get in a cycle of worry that leads to more disrupted sleep. Congratulations, you have proven you are human! You have successfully gotten in the way of a major physiological drive. And I'm sorry about that. The good news is that you can also get out of the way if you know what to look for.

My goal for this book is not to train you to manage a sleep disorder or insomnia. My goal is to help you develop the habits in your daily life that will make it easier to get back to healthy sleep, especially when you've had a bad night, or two or three. You will experience stress, frustration, challenges, and hurdles in your life because, as Buddhists point out, living is suffering. But choosing to focus on what we can control can help us get back to better living and better sleep. If you are suffering from a sleep disorder or insomnia, talk to your primary care physician or seek out a sleep professional—most sleep disorders are very treatable, so the time you delay seeking treatment is time you are missing out.

## EXCEPTIONS

Everyone sleeps and everyone is human, and these tips are for the humans who sleep. However, there are reasons these ideas will be especially challenging for some and won't work for others. If you can change the items on this list that fit you, my tips will be easier for you to use.

1. **You perform shift work.**
   Most of my suggestions are based on living as a diurnal (not nocturnal) human—that is, someone who is alert in the day and sleeps at night. We are all engineered to operate as diurnal animals, no matter how much of a night owl you

are. If you are a shift worker, some of this book will still apply to you but not all of it.

While I am on the subject, if you are a shift worker, I hope you can consider transitioning your work into non-shift work. There is ample evidence that long-term shift work is very hard on your health. I have tremendous respect for the health care workers, emergency services providers, and military members, not to mention the plumbers and electricians, who perform essential duties while on shift work. I encourage all of you to move to day-shift work permanently when you are able and let others take the overnight work. This will be the first step toward better sleep and health.

2. **You fall into the Class III obesity category.**
It's a fact that as our modern lives have become less physical, as healthy foods become harder to acquire while unhealthy foods are inexpensive and plentiful, and as our routines become more sedentary, our bodies have become less physically fit. You are a person worthy of great care and kindness, and I am glad you are seeking help for your sleep!

More people are living with Class III obesity (a BMI of 40 or greater, or 35 or greater with obesity-related health problems) than ever in the history of humans. Living with Class III obesity means your body is fighting to stay alive. One of the strongest indicators for obstructive sleep apnea (OSA) is Class III obesity. Estimates in 2019 from researcher Adam Benjafield's team suggest that about 936 million adults globally live with OSA, most of them undiagnosed. The United States ranks second highest in prevalence.[1] Your chances of heart attack, stroke, diabetes, and early death all increase drastically when you have OSA. Treatment of OSA is effective, but for some people, one of the most effective ways to cure OSA is weight loss.

If you struggle with Class III obesity, talk to your primary care provider about getting help. But don't stop there—talk to your family and your friends, anyone who you believe will support you in attaining a healthier weight. Having accountability buddies is often the most crucial aspect of making any major change.

If you are obese, the suggestions in this book will apply to you, and they will be easier to follow when your body is struggling less to breathe during your night of sleep.

3. **You have a substance addiction (e.g., opioids, alcohol, or stimulants like Adderall) that prevents you from practicing some of the recommendations.**
If you need help with ending an addiction, please seek professional help. If you are concerned that your chronic medical or physical illness isn't being treated effectively, please seek additional resources. Excellent providers are available; if you find yourself stuck with someone who doesn't seem to know how to help you, keep looking. If you got a bad haircut, would you go back to the same person for another haircut?

Addiction issues can be strongly connected to sleep challenges. Each of you has your own challenges, and some of you have inspired me to write a book. Again, portions of this book will still apply to you, but these recommendations will be easier to use and more meaningful when you are on the other side of your addiction.

4. **You are the caretaker for someone who often needs assistance overnight.**
   You deserve recognition. Whether you are caring for an infant, a toddler, or the special needs of your child, your parent, or another loved one, you may not be in control of your schedule and your sleep. I see you, and I appreciate what you do.
   Some of this book may be difficult for you to apply to your lifestyle, but all of it is likely to be relevant to you. You can probably use many aspects of these suggestions now and can use the intentions behind these ideas to better your sleep.

## HOW DID WE GET HERE?

### Why Your Sleep Isn't What It Could Be

#### TL;DR

In the beginning of time, it was dark. Then there was light. About 4.54 billion years later, our ancestors started adding to the light by making fire. *Homo sapiens* only showed up recently, about 300,000 years ago. It's been just over 100 years that we humans have been creating light that is inexpensive, very bright, and easily accessible. Sure, there was insomnia before that, but not nearly as advanced and impressive as our modern insomnia. Insomnia is likely another invention of modern humanity.

Let me expand on that idea. Where I live, people get impressed with one-hundred-year-old buildings. I do too. It's interesting to see how things were built and considered state of the art a century ago. Things have really changed in one hundred years. We now have heating, cooling, lighting, comfortable seating, many carpeting options, and so much more. It's the evolution of modern life. Rarely has there been a period in history with such an explosion of products that made life more comfortable (think air conditioning instead of sweltering), safer (think vaccines instead of being disabled by polio), and easier (think driving to the store instead of walking or pulling a mule). As much as the advancements have made things easier for us, could it be that they have also made sleep more difficult?

## Circadian Rhythms: Keeping Us on Track for 300,000 Years

In the last million years, humans (*Homo sapiens*) evolved from *Homo neanderthalensis*, *Homo heidelbergensis*, and *Homo erectus*. These species evolved from other hominins over several million years before that. And even before that, our ancestors' ancestors were evolving for millions of years. A few things were consistent across those millions of years. The sunlight and the dark were consistent. The days lasted right around twenty-four hours for all of those last several million years—essentially the same as today.

Your parents may have told you that you are a special person, and you are to some degree, but everyone's brain and body are programmed to work on the same twenty-four-hour cycle that is determined by the cycle of night and day. That twenty-four-hour internal cycle is called our circadian rhythm (that's Latin for "about [*circa*] a day [*dian*]") or chronobiology.

We can expect that those ancestors of ours were spending most of their days awake and most of their nights sleeping while it was dark. Our bodies and brains evolved an internal biological clock to manage our days and nights in ways that made the most sense. And we pass this chronobiological clock to our offspring through our genes.

As animals at the top or close to the top of the food chain (I'm talking about us humans), it was relatively safe for us to sleep at night—we were unlikely to be attacked by animals or rival humans while we were sleeping. Humans function better in the day, and that made us diurnal (not nocturnal). Like all diurnal animals, daily functioning is driven by a complicated series of neurochemical transactions. These include the times of day we are hungry, tired, most alert, need to use the bathroom, as well as the times of day we are most resistant to viruses and so many other things.

One way you can see the human circadian rhythm or chronobiology play out is by bathroom use. Research on large groups of people reported on by Timothy Hibberd and his team in 2023 has shown that the average time of day when the greatest number of humans empty their bowels is between 7:00 a.m. and 9:00 a.m.[2] Our circadian rhythms encourage lots of us to get to the bathroom at right around 8:30 a.m. Next time you are in a large group between the hours of 8:00 a.m. and 9:00 a.m., take notice of how many people need to leave the group to use the washroom during that period. Then immediately try to forget. This is not especially fun information to have. But it demonstrates the power of the human circadian rhythm well. Not everyone will use the bathroom at the same time because evolution doesn't want us to do that. But some people will, and more of them during that hour than at any other hour of the day.

## Why Do Some of Us Prefer Morning and Others Evening?

Some of you are reading this and thinking, "No way are we all the same. I can stay up until 2:00 a.m. and am at my best around midnight, but I can't wake up before 8:00 a.m., while my friend is up every day at 7:00 a.m., no matter how late he was up the previous night."

While all of us are diurnal (not nocturnal), like most things with human genetics, chronobiology isn't rigid. Let's think about those differences.

Another way that human evolution is likely to have helped humans is by fostering a preference for mornings or evenings. In 2017, David Samson and his team of genetic and chronobiologic researchers proposed the concept that these preferences developed as a method of sentinel behavior to protect our group from predators, like a night watch.[3] Although we were at or near the top of the food chain for the last million years, we did have enemies and predators (many of which looked a lot like us). Keeping watch over the group would be an important technique for maintaining safety in any group. If evolution could encourage some of us to prefer a later bedtime while others prefer an early wake time, we would have a watch-person most of the night.

One feature of humans today is that if you gather a group of thirty or forty of us together, about the same size as most human groups over the last million years, you'll find a few group members are naturally "night owls," and a few are naturally "morning larks." In addition, Mary Carskadon's lifetime of research demonstrates that between starting puberty and our mid-twenties, young adults have a neurochemical preference for a bedtime about two hours later than other adults,[4] making the overnight safety watch more robust with those who are healthiest to take watch.

Evolution likely preferred humans who lived in groups large enough to have some night owls and some morning larks. A group would also have been safer with enough young adults to keep watch overnight and early in the morning because they preferred to be awake at those times.

Our bodies fine-tuned a twenty-four-hour sleep-and-wake cycle during the last three hundred thousand years. When humans lived with the sun but without much artificial light, things related to sleeping and waking were simple. There was a lot to do during the day: finding food, finding safe places to sleep and rest, telling jokes, and so on. It was a busy life. When the sun went down, not much else could be done. You could maybe work on a new joke or song, make a pass at the attractive humanoid you've been smiling at all day, or groom your friend to help get rid of their ticks or lice. Eventually, sleep would come.

In the winter months, and the further north one lives, the longer darkness lasts at night. If you live in Toronto or Calgary, you experience an extended nighttime darkness that someone who lives in Houston doesn't. If you and your family were living ten thousand years ago and in a colder climate, as winter approached you might be starting to migrate south. Meanwhile your pre-bedtime routine probably began by about 6:00 p.m. The sun might not be visible for the next thirteen hours. You aren't going to sleep thirteen hours, are you? You are going to sleep for a while, wake up for a while, then probably drift off and sleep or rest some more. It is too dangerous to walk around in the dark and too expensive to have a lamp, torch, or fire burning all night. Instead, you wait for the sun to come up. This is a recipe for getting enough sleep—have plenty of opportunity and nothing else to do.

There is evidence in writing from a few hundred years ago that this style of "first sleep" and "second sleep," or splitting the night into two distinct sleep phases, was still common, according to Niall Boyce. It makes sense because even as recently as the 1800s,[5] getting light by burning a candle or lamp, manure, coal, or wood was an expensive thing to do. People saved their money and stayed in bed.

### FAQ TO GO DEEP ON SLEEP: Should I sleep like a jaguar?

My roommate in college read about the sleeping habits of jaguars and started sleeping the same way. He couldn't keep it up for long. Why is that?

I was making a presentation decades ago when someone pressed me to explain the practicalities of being diurnal. He explained that his college roommate read about the sleeping habits of jaguars and tried sleeping the same way. It didn't take long for his roommate to give up, but now I was being asked why that would be. At first, I assumed he was just pranking me. At the same time, I was presenting to a roomful of physicians and nurses, and I knew this guy was a physician. So I asked him, "Was your college roommate a jaguar?" Laughter filled the room, not because I'm so funny, but probably because everyone else was wondering why this doctor asked such a ridiculous question.

But let's take this question at face value and stop judging this misunderstood physician—let's call him Dr. Jaguar. I write a lot in this book about circadian rhythms, but more specifically, what I'm writing about are the circadian rhythms of humans, assuming that most of my readers will be human. Those readers who aren't human should call me because I'd like to meet a dog, cat, dolphin, or whatever who is so interested in sleep that they've read this far in this book.

Back to the point. Dr. Jaguar couldn't maintain the sleep habits of an actual jaguar because it isn't human. Jaguars are crepuscular, meaning they are most active at dawn and dusk (great times for hunting), and they sleep in smaller bursts. On the other hand, jaguars sleep between ten and eleven hours per day. Dr. Jaguar was enticed by the idea that maybe he could sleep three to four hours here and there and maintain a high quality of life (like a jaguar?). What he didn't account for is that jaguars sleep three to four hours at a time, three to four times per day. Most college students don't have that kind of time to dedicate to being asleep. Honestly, I don't know any human who does.

In addition, humans are built to be diurnal, not crepuscular, meaning our brains want us to be active in daytime and to rest at nighttime. While some humans enjoy the late nights more than mornings and vice versa, all humans are built to rest overnight and be alert in the day. Finally, Dr. Jaguar may never have developed the ability to sleep in trees, which is sort of an essential jaguar thing.

The surprising real point I got to is to answer the question of whether you should let your dog or cat sleep in bed with you. While the answer varies based on several factors, my recommendation is not to allow a new dog, cat, puppy, or kitten in bed with you. As cold and heartless as this sounds, your sleep is very different from a puppy's or a kitten's. And if you've rescued an older dog or cat, you simply don't know one another well enough to sleep soundly in a bed together right away.

More to the point, the circadian rhythms of dogs and cats are quite different from those of humans. If you've ever tried to nap every time your cat tried to nap, you'll know what I mean. Both dogs and cats sleep far more than humans do, and like jaguars, they do it in smaller bursts than humans do. So, while it's cute, cuddly, and comfortable to fall asleep with your pet, at some point in the next few hours they will be up, walking around, scratching, burrowing between your legs, messing with your hair, or just walking around the house in a way that isn't conducive to human sleep. You can't expect them to consider your sleep needs; you are in charge of that.

## LET THERE BE (CHEAP, ACCESSIBLE) LIGHT

In the late 1800s Thomas Edison reinvented the light bulb with a filament that would last a good long time. According to Sara Cottle's[6] and Efosa Ojomo's[7] reviews, parts of Manhattan had electric lights in 1892, but it would be more than thirty years before half of the homes in the US had electric lights. By 1949, 90% of US homes had electricity. And by 1960, nearly all homes had electricity. Imagine that: It's only been four generations since your relatives lived without electricity or lights in their home. And if your relatives lived on a farm in the early 1900s, like mine did, it's probably been less than four generations, or less than one hundred years, that Americans have enjoyed artificial light in their homes.

In one of my presentations with college students, I talked about these changes. A student asked me if human brains hadn't simply evolved since Edison's lightbulb so that we are able to deal with the decreased amount of darkness in our lives. I asked him to look at his pinky and consider how long evolution has been working on getting rid of human pinkies and then consider whether one hundred years is enough for evolution to manage the additional light from light bulbs. While some adaptive evolutionary steps happen as quickly as seven or eight generations for lizards and snow voles, it seems likely that changes to the chronobiology of humans will take far longer. In addition, humans are not all getting a uniform change to their light input, which means evolutionary change is unlikely to be happening.

Let me put this in perspective: For *hundreds of thousands of years*, human brains relied on sunlight to mark days and darkness to mark nights. Beautiful, intricately built circadian rhythms were developed that run in natural response to the light and dark, as well as the daily activities of each of us. There was fire, but fire took a lot of effort and resources to maintain throughout the dark nights. Then, in the blink of an evolutionary eye, humans had access to light bulbs, making it possible to have inexpensive, bright light twenty-four hours a day. What could go wrong?

The answer, which is probably what brought you to this book in the first place, is problems sleeping and regulating your day and night routines. When your brain no longer has a consistent daylight/darkness pattern, it becomes more difficult for it to help you get to sleep and wake up. To take this one step further, for decades, we were only dealing with electric lights. Sure, lightbulbs made it easier to stay up late doing things, but the things we were doing in the evenings back in the 1940s and early 1950s were straightforward. This was the era of cribbage, bridge, poker, and late-night games like charades and Scrabble. There were other distractions, including the radio, recorded music on the hi-fi, and more access to cars to take us places anytime, day or night, but the world of electronic entertainment was just about to begin.

## FIRST, LIGHT. THEN, ENTERTAINMENT

Then came the rapid flood of electronic advancements, from television to Nintendo, from the late 1950s to the end of the 1990s. It was one new gadget after another. When Pong came out in the late 1970s, it seemed clear that we were on the precipice of something major. Being able to play that game at home on our own TV was nothing short of amazing to my brother and me in the late 1970s. Home gaming systems were on their way next with the Atari 2600 and game cartridges. Fast-forward fifty years and games are still played similarly—at home, on a personal device with friends. But everything else about gaming has changed. I'm getting ahead of myself, though.

From the beginning of television, there were decades when programming ended somewhere between 10:30 p.m. and midnight every night of the week. It's hard to imagine now, but before cable television there would be static on every station for hours overnight. There was a "nothing to see here, move along" situation late at night. Steve Martin, on his "Let's Get Small" comedy album in the 1970s, had a joke about how important he was and how busy he was. "I've got a lot of important things to do. Are you kidding? A guy like me without important things to do? [long pause] What time does TV go off?"[8]

When CNN and twenty-four-hour news hit the airwaves, things began to change. Cable television was still in its infancy in 1980, but the pathway was built for news coverage, and then everything else on television, to be aired every hour of the day. In essence, when households transitioned from using their TV antennae to cable television, they invited twenty-four-hour programming into their homes, which has never let up. This was in the 1980s for most households, and the following decade for most of the rest.

Do you know someone who has a TV in their bedroom? Do you know someone who watches TV in bed? Do you know people who keep the TV on all night while they sleep? These activities didn't happen before the 1980s because without cable television, there literally wasn't anything to watch after bedtime.

Why am I writing about TVs and cable news in a book about sleep? Because TV viewing late in the evening, especially the distressing or cliff-hanger shows, became a new reason for having a bad night of sleep, or a series of them. And because cable television is a moving target, it reinvents itself every few years with more options. Cable TV has developed over the decades from a few extra channels in the 1980s to hundreds of (mostly unwatched) channels and several pay services like Netflix and Hulu with infinite content available on demand anytime. I haven't even mentioned the internet and social media yet. A reinvented entertainment system creates new ways to be engaged and entertained again and again. It's great for entertaining you but is not so great for your rest.

## ENTERTAINMENT AND SLEEP DEPRIVATION

Don't get me wrong, I love Netflix, and I really enjoy watching professional cycling on Peacock, college basketball on ESPN+, and *Zelda* on my Switch. I enjoy the developments in technology and entertainment; my goal here is to help you be aware of the pitfalls.

Let me bring this together for you. As long as science has been studying sleep, it has also been studying the limits of sleep deprivation and how fatigue affects performance. You can imagine why the military would be interested in these concepts, but so are professional athletes, production management, the Department of Transportation, the Federal Aviation Administration, the Highway Safety Commission, and so on.

For many years, sleep researchers have paid healthy adults to stay awake in their labs as long as possible so that their ability to perform tasks could be measured at various stages of fatigue and sleep deprivation. Researchers would not allow caffeine or stimulant medications to be used to boost alertness, but they would allow just about anything else. Before cable television, TV wasn't helpful because programming ended at the end of the evening. Randy Gardner stayed awake for hundreds of hours mostly through playing ping pong and pinball.[9]

Why were ping pong and pinball so effective? Let's compare ping pong to reading a book or listening to music. Both use brain power and are engaging. But ping pong is fast-moving, and the action changes based on the actions of the player in real time. You can't zone out playing ping pong and play well. One aspect that helps people stay awake is doing something active where your actions have immediate implications to the outcome. Reading and listening to music don't do this.

Let's fast-forward half a century. What activities would you expect participants to be doing these days while trying to stay awake without substances? Did you guess video games? Then you are right. The ping pong and pinball of the 1960s are now *The Legend of Zelda* and *Fortnite*. To be honest, the researchers will probably let you bring whatever game you enjoy playing to the lab, not just the janky pinball machine they got on loan from the student lounge, because they want you to succeed in staying awake. Letting you play what you want to play will encourage you to stay awake longer. The same principles are at work here—active games, where your actions have real-time consequences and frequent or constant interactivity with the game, keep the brain alert.

Our brains love this sort of activity. It's one of the reasons why video games are so enticing. What else can you do in your life where you design and decide every action, and you can constantly interact with the world around you with significant consequences for hours at a time? And right now, you probably have a few of these beautifully designed video games within arm's reach, even if you are in the bathroom. That's because all the game engineering that has gone into the high-end video games on expensive consoles has also gone into the free games you download on your smartphone. From the bright colors to the quick action, the differences are minimal, and the effect smartphone games have on your brain is the same.

If you could fill a room with engineers, programmers, brain scientists, and graphic artists and ask them to build a product that would help people stay awake for long hours while still being productive with their product, I'm not sure it would look much different from the gaming we have today. Modern video games on your phone and Xbox are graphically realistic, interactive at a speed we experience as equal to or even faster than real life, and only getting better at these aspects every year (every month?) as technology improves. Neurologically, our dopamine receptors are engaged repetitively, and while playing games we get a dopamine response that feels great and makes us want to keep coming back for more.

If you are reading this section and congratulating yourself because you aren't playing video games, I have some bad news for you. The same technology that makes modern video games so engaging is being used in places you spend your time, too. *Candy Crush* and phone games have the same technology, but so does YouTube, TikTok, your news app, pornography, and your online shopping. From the perspective of marketers and industry, why wouldn't they try to keep you on their site longer? They use all the techniques that maximize your brain chemistry to prolong your visit. It's good business sense and terrible for humans in the long run.

## Your Brain on Games

Here's another way to think about modern gaming, TikTok, and the like. Imagine someone who was alive long ago was reincarnated and landed in a modern living room. Let's call your visitor Dudley. It doesn't matter to me if Dudley is from 1910, 1725, or 440 BC. (Spoiler alert: That's because Dudley's brain hasn't evolved much since then). After Dudley gets over the astonishment of modern furniture and lighting, you are ready to introduce him to the TikTok and Instagram apps. No need to explain the interface, really, just how to scroll, watch videos, and turn on the sound. Once Dudley is ready for a break from the cat videos, people falling off things, and makeup tutorials, it's time to take things up to the next level: modern video games. You download *Candy Crush* or *Royal Kingdom*, or *Roblox* or *Call of Duty* mobile. You teach Dudley how to play and come back five hours later with something to eat because all this gaming has made Dudley hungry.

Dudley is having the same reaction to the apps and to the games that each of us has. It's probably more thrilling for him because he is from 1745, but once the thrill is over, his brain reacts the same as ours does because evolutionarily our brains haven't changed. When we first use these games, our brains are thrilled, literally. We dream about moving those colored blocks around and how to run from or fight the bad guys while we sleep. Our brains have difficulty sitting around and reading a book, listening to a lecture, or even watching a standard TV show without doing some phone checking because our brain knows there is something far more engaging with just the click of a button or a tap of an icon. And right behind that button or icon is an endless supply of dopamine and instant gratification.

Dudley's brain is built just like your brain. Whether he lived one hundred or two thousand years ago, he responds to engagement and dopamine boosts the same.

Evolution takes much longer than a few decades to make significant changes. And these changes to our lives are brand new. From an evolutionary perspective, the beginning of light bulbs, television, TikTok, and video games has happened in the blink of an eye.

Why spend so much time telling you about this? Because lights and entertainment have an impact on your ability to sleep at night and be awake in the day. Because we are surrounded by TV, social media, shopping, pornography, and video games (the big ones and the little ones on your phone). Because we are already so accustomed to their role in our lives that most people, especially those born after 2005, think of them as normal.

I'm not going to tell you to end your use of all your devices and accounts, although there are some compelling reasons to do so. But since you are reading for some good ways to improve your chances of having better, healthier sleep, let me use this opportunity to give you some ideas for changing your use of entertainment and lighting to encourage better sleep.

It's a long path from a million years ago but a short hop from when light bulbs became inexpensive and used everywhere. And in the last fifty years the leaps in technology have made it challenging for our bodies and our brains to know when it's time to settle down for a good night of sleep. For some, technology has made it nearly impossible to get a good night of sleep.

## MORE REASONS NOT TO SLEEP WELL

Technology offers more than enough reasons to have difficulty with sleep, right? Yes, *and* the world offers additional opportunities to develop poor sleep. The way we live indoors, the billion-dollar "Sleep Better Now!" industry encouraging us to buy unnecessary things to make us sleepier, and the way we each handle these three facts of life make the struggle real. Let me talk you through each of those before I launch into my top tips for better sleep and better living.

### We Had Help Getting Here: The Sleep Better Now! Industry

At the end of the day and the end of this book, how you handle your sleep is personal. You make the decisions about your daily activities, your sleeping activities, and how you think about the nights when you sleep poorly. You have power over all the ways you can approach these aspects of your life. And as you've already learned, sleep is an essential drive for humans.

Why is it that so many of us struggle with our sleep when sleep is built into our biology? We don't struggle to drink water when we are thirsty. So why do we struggle to sleep when we are exhausted?

There are many reasons. Our lifestyle in the modern twenty-first century doesn't align well with our chronobiology: all the time indoors, all the social media and streaming content that we can look at twenty-four hours a day, and so on. These things don't help. According to Charles Matthews' research group,[10] Americans spend half their waking hours sitting, and according to the Environmental Protection Agency[11] and the Occupational Safety and Health Administration,[12] Americans spend about 90% of their time indoors or in a vehicle. Our bodies aren't built for this lifestyle.

There is another, more insidious problem that is part of the world we live in. This problem is all around us as well. It is well funded and well advertised. In fact, that's a major part of the issue: The problem is effectively marketed as providing helpful, meaningful products to promote sleep. I'm talking about the *Sleep Better Now!* industry. Socks to help us sleep more, skin creams to deepen our sleep, sound machines, special mattresses, sheets, pajamas, bedroom lights, sunglasses, sleep trackers, supplements, and pharmaceuticals . . . the list goes on and on. There is a multi-billion-dollar-per-year industry built to sell you things related to improving your sleep.

I understand the irony of my telling you this while you are holding a book in your hands that you purchased to help improve your sleep. What's different is that my goal with this book is to help you sleep better without the help of the *Sleep Better Now!* industry. I want to help you do it by relearning how to use what your body and brain are built for—so you can sleep better over the long run. I also want you to be able to look at the advertisements and promotions that inundate us and decide what you do and don't need. (Spoiler alert: There isn't anything being sold that you need.) And then I will teach you to maximize your circadian rhythms essentially without the help of any products or supplements.

Let me explain this differently. Everyone has a bad night of sleep from time to time. Most adults struggle with sleep a couple of nights every month. That is normal. When it is you lying awake at three o'clock in the morning with nothing to do, maybe you open your phone and scroll Instagram and TikTok. What advertisements do you see at that time of day? You see more ads for *Sleep Better Now!* Suddenly you think you may be the only person awake at that hour, and you must be doing something wrong.

Maybe you decide to buy the perfect pillow or the new supplement that some influencer, athlete, or neuroscientist is recommending for sleeping like a baby. Then you wait for the pillow or supplement to arrive while raising your expectations for how your sleep is going to improve once you have this item, making it a bit harder to sleep while you are waiting—you know you have been missing out on this "essential" aspect of good sleep. Once it arrives you excitedly get in bed for the new experience.

Maybe you luck out, and it is helpful for your sleep (congrats!). This is the new you, and you tell your friends about it so they can have *Sleep Better Now!* too. You are pleased with your purchase and look forward to sleep.

Then something happens. Down the road a week, or a month, you have a bad night of sleep again. Maybe you understand what caused it, or maybe not. Either way, one bad night is followed by another. Next thing you know you are awake at three o'clock in the morning, scrolling Instagram or TikTok and getting more targeted advertisements for *Sleep Better Now!* products and wondering if you bought the wrong product last time—maybe you need this new product. After all, a super healthy athlete endorsed it, and they must sleep well. And then you decide to buy the product, and the cycle begins again.

This happens every day of the year. It's happening right now while you read this. There are products for every aspect of your sleep that you can purchase and have in your home this week. And there are people making money off your concerns and fears about sleep with nothing more than a product and some vague sense that it could be helpful. And they will continue to make that money because people will continue to wonder if that product could be the one thing that puts them over the top to great sleep.

You don't really need any of those products to sleep well. Most likely you used to sleep just fine without that pillow, supplement, or special sheets. Am I right? Even if you have always had difficulty sleeping, you are unlikely to need specialty items for sleeping. Humans have been sleeping, mostly well, for hundreds of thousands of years—keep that in mind. Also, humans have probably always had bad nights of sleep here and there. That's normal, too. And humans like to try new things to improve parts of their lives that are important to them. They also prefer to buy something or take a supplement more than they like to make lifestyle changes that are somewhat unpleasant. I'm no different and I know better. Take some solace in that.

You don't need a special or expensive pillow or mattress to sleep well; that much is true. But since this is a question I get often, let's talk about it. Because while the bedding industry often overpromises, there are still some practical things worth knowing.

### The Bedding Industry Has a Product for You!

Foam, pillow top, cooling/heating, automatic head raising, split sides, firm, soft, medium, for side-sleepers, for back-sleepers, and so on, and so on. They appeal to our need for something better, something that will make those challenges at night easier. Sometimes they are right—they can help us sleep better. Sometimes they are just marketing and trying to sell you something you don't need. How are you to know the difference?

I am not an expert in bedding or pillows. I am a sleep psychologist. Let's start there. Do I have opinions based on being a sleep psychologist? I certainly do! Let's air them out.

First and foremost, humans sleep. Remember that no matter what you sleep on, or how much money you spend, most humans throughout history slept on much less and generally slept fine. There are billions of people right now who will sleep on little more than a pad tonight. And they will sleep fine. Human bodies can adjust to just about anything, and the drive for sleep is so strong that your body will, over time, adapt to your bedding.

Now that you don't have to worry about spending top dollar, are there reasons to consider specialty bedding? Sure.

Is your mattress more than ten years old? It's time to replace it. Mattresses are not lifetime objects. You spend hours lying there every night, so respect yourself and your sleep and find a new mattress.

How old is your pillow? Five years is my limit. Remember those nights when you woke up drooling on your pillow? There are only so many drooling nights and subsequent pillow washings that your pillow can be expected to tolerate before breaking down into less than what it was designed to be.

There are other reasons to update or pay close attention to your bedding: Chronic pain or injury is at the top of the list. Many clients I've worked with have chronic back pain for one reason or another. A firm mattress is generally better for managing back pain. This is similar for chronic neck pain and pillows. Firm is generally better.

Do you and your partner share a bed and have vastly different preferences for mattress firmness? I think the bedding industry did couples a massive favor when they introduced mattresses that accommodate different firmness preferences for the left and right sides of the bed. It's been a huge win in my household.

Do you and your partner share a bed and have vastly different preferences for covers or temperature while sleeping? Do you like to sleep with five blankets, while they like to sleep under one blanket with their feet sticking out because they are so hot? One of the best developments in the last several years in the world of bedding and happy couples has been the creation of temperature-controlled bedding (hot and cold). This is best done with the use of water-filled tubes that run through a removable mattress cover and cycle through a device that heats or cools the water outside the bed. These devices are expensive, but I've never met someone who used one and didn't find it to be a game changer.

What's the downside of having the pillow, mattress, or blankets that are exactly right for you? Once you get used to sleeping in a bed that is just right for you, leaving home and sleeping in a different bed means you are going to experience a less personal—and most likely less comfortable—bedding experience. Is that the end of the world? No. You may not sleep as well away from home, but you are traveling for a reason, right? Lean into the reasons for being where you are and appreciate the sleep you get. It will feel amazing to return to your curated sleep environment when you return home. And if it's just a pillow that makes all the difference, consider whether it's worth traveling with your pillow!

Last word on this—bedding is personal. The salesperson in your mattress store and online will try to convince you that their product is the best ever for you and everyone you know. Here's the secret: No one can tell you absolutely what will work for you in the realm of pillows, mattresses, or blankets. It's a bit like food—some foods, like pizza, most people like, and some foods, like lima beans, are more of an acquired taste. Even among pizza lovers, everyone has their favorite, and few agree. That's okay; you can all be right because it's your pizza. Think of your mattress and pillows similarly. Just because the salesperson or your coworker knows the best mattress in the world that you are going to absolutely love, trust your own experience. Most mattress companies offer risk-free ninety-night trials. Take them up on this and don't be bashful about returning a mattress that isn't working for you.

### What About Sleep Medications?

Before we move on, I want to address sleep medications: from antihistamines to prescription-only medications designed specifically to help you sleep. For most people, there is little more convincing than having their own doctor talk to them about sleep medications. One problem with this is that, according to Jodi Mindell's investigation of medical schools in twelve countries, on average, medical schools provide about 2.5 hours of training on sleep disorders. About half that time is spent on obstructive sleep apnea (OSA), which is helpful if you have OSA. Twenty-seven percent of the schools who responded reported their school did not provide sleep education at all. In the United States and Canada, the average amount of time spend on sleep education was 3 hours.[13]

Most people see their primary care physician for insomnia (which can mask OSA sometimes) and are often prescribed a medication for insomnia. Fortunately, most physicians trained since 2010 have been trained to understand that the medications designed for sleep are short-term solutions and rarely address underlying sleep problems. The physicians trained more recently have heard that the first-line treatment for insomnia is cognitive behavioral therapy for insomnia (CBTI), not medications. Unfortunately, practitioners who are good at using CBTI are often hard to find and often have long waiting lists.

There are times when sleep medications are a good idea and when I fully support their use. These are the times in life when a person can't sleep and there is a specific, easily identified, time-limited reason for using a medication. Maybe it's a very important presentation at a conference or to the board of trustees; maybe your partner or child is having surgery in two weeks, and you are very concerned about how it goes. Maybe there is a positive reason that brings stress, like next week you are moving to a new city to start a new job with a person you really love, and all the exciting changes are making it impossible to sleep.

These are all good reasons to speak with your primary care physician about a short-term sleep medication. But be careful—it's tempting to ask for a refill of that prescription and to continue taking it. I have learned from years of working with my clients that even the sleep medications that were amazingly effective at the beginning lose their effectiveness over time. And when you have come to rely on a medication to help you sleep, it can be devastating when it no longer does its job.

### The Risks of the Z-Drugs

When medications like Ambien (Lunesta, Sonata, Edluar, and Imovane) were initially released in the early 1990s, there was a hushed expectation that there might never be insomnia again. As a group, these drugs are referred to as the *Z-drugs* since the letter Z is part of most of their generic names (eszopiclone, zaleplon, and zolpidem). These drugs target your GABA production and help you feel calmer. There is a risk for addiction, but in the early days these drugs were approved for prolonged use, and many physicians became comfortable with prescribing them for months, years, or indefinitely.

Instead of curing insomnia, we now have millions of Americans taking a medication nightly that many of them believe "doesn't help me sleep anymore, but if I stop taking it, I won't sleep at all." I have a biased sample of clientele who struggle with sleep, but even among people I meet casually this refrain is common.

After several years of these medications being prescribed, emergency department physicians across the country noticed a new trend in the patients they were seeing overnight. These were people who injured themselves while under the influence of a Z-drug. In fact, in a statement published by the Substance Abuse and Mental Health Services Administration, the number of Ambien-related emergency department visits increased 220% from just over six thousand visits in 2005 to over nineteen thousand in 2010.[14]

Eventually, it was understood that these people were experiencing a side effect of a Z-drug called *complex sleep behaviors*. At first glance, they look like someone sleepwalking—moving around and doing things with vague or little purpose to the nonsleeping viewer. They are clearly not awake. The difference is that with complex sleep behaviors, the activities are far more complex than with sleepwalking.

Complex sleep behaviors, on the other hand, are generally activities that the sleeper often does without much thought during the day but required weeks or years to develop. They are more likely to include manipulating an object effectively (think of using kitchen items or changing clothes). Complex sleep behaviors include walking, taking other medications, riding the bus to work, cooking, and even driving. The sleeper will sometimes have a vague memory of their activities but not much more than that.

Years ago, I was working with a client named Ahmed who wanted to stop taking Ambien nightly but was very fearful that he would "never sleep again." Ironically, after taking Ambien he couldn't fall asleep for ninety minutes (the first sign the medication was no longer working), but on a night when he just went without it, he reported getting no sleep at all. We were in the process of getting started with CBTI when Ahmed came to our third session to tell me he had a weird experience and thought I should know about it. He explained that when he woke up that morning, he found a receipt from 7-Eleven on his nightstand showing he bought cigarettes, his typical brand. Also, on his nightstand were the butts of three cigarettes he smoked.

Working backward, Ahmed put the pieces together. He took his Ambien before bed at about 11:30 p.m. He got in bed and remembered struggling to fall asleep, as usual, likely drifting off around 1:00 a.m. The receipt he found shows he made his purchase of cigarettes at 2:15 a.m. at a 7-Eleven where he often buys cigarettes. To do so, he needed to get in his car, drive to 7-Eleven, make the purchase, get back in his car, and drive home—all behaviors he does while awake without thinking much about it. At this point, he was pretty freaked out. He realized that he was driving while asleep, or if he was awake, it wasn't awake enough to remember. But the last piece of the puzzle, and the next most frightening aspect of his experience, is that he smoked three cigarettes while in bed—something he would never do intentionally because of the risk of falling asleep while smoking and catching his bed on fire. He finally had clear motivation to cease his Ambien.

While some of the stories are innocuous or funny, many are frightening, like Ahmed's, and tragic. In 2019, the FDA issued a black box warning for Ambien due to reports of complex sleep behaviors that led to people being burned, overdosing, wandering outside in extreme cold, shooting themselves with firearms, and thousands of falls and other accidents (U.S. Food and Drug Administration, 2019).[15]

This is now a known side effect of the Z-drugs (not just Ambien), and there is no way of knowing whether a person will experience this side effect. For one person, complex sleep behaviors might never happen; for others, they could occur after the first dose of a Z-drug—or they could show up one night after years of taking a Z-drug with no side effects, as was the case for Ahmed. While it's true that not everyone who takes a Z-drug will experience complex sleep behaviors, it is also true that there are probably many times more experiences of these behaviors that are never reported because the sleeper doesn't remember them and has no injury or receipt from 7-Eleven. They are hard to capture in a drug trial because they occur randomly (as far as we can tell), and drug trials don't last long enough to effectively capture them.

Bottom line: If your friend takes a Z-drug and is boiling potatoes in the middle of the night, it may seem funny at the time. But this is a serious side effect of a strong medication that has led to accidental overdose, self-inflicted gunshots, injury, and death. Even a single experience of complex sleep behaviors is reason enough to stop taking a Z-drug.

My recommendation: After an experience like this, call your prescribing physician and let them know you have had the side effect of complex sleep behaviors and you need to stop taking the Z-drug immediately. Your physician may not know about complex sleep behaviors, but you know enough. If you have a medical reason to need some medication for sleep, ask your doctor to consider something that isn't in the Z-drug category.

### What Supplements Do You Recommend for Sleep?

I get this question quite a bit. And it's a short answer: I don't recommend any supplements for sleep.

What I do recommend is a healthy, nutritious diet with plenty of fresh foods eaten in reasonable portions. And get outside to take advantage of the vitamin D that the sun is giving you every day. The vitamin D and helpful blue light from the sun come through during daylight hours, even when it's raining.

If your physician reads your blood test results and determines you need a supplement, follow those directions.

If you watch a TikTok video that says one supplement, or blend of supplements, cured their insomnia, do not assume it's accurate or true. Talk about it with your primary care physician before trying.

While we are here, I want to say two things about your melatonin use. First, you are probably taking too much of it, a 4 mg dose is recommended for help falling asleep. Second, if you live in the United States, the amount of melatonin printed on the bottle is quite possibly wildly different from the amount of actual melatonin inside the tablet or gummy. This is the result when supplements like melatonin are not regulated by the Federal Drug Administration (FDA). Two research studies have shown the tested amounts of melatonin to be as little as 78% less and as much as 486% more than what is printed on the bottle.[16]

## We Are Here—Let's Get Better

Let's review, shall we? Today, millions of people struggle with sleep for many reasons. Living in the twenty-first century is amazing with our miraculous health care systems, our ability to access healthy foods easily, and our technological advances. It also makes activities our bodies did naturally for millennia more difficult.

We spend far more time indoors and away from the sunlight, which trains and resets our internal circadian clocks naturally. Our jobs and our free time tend to bring us indoors rather than living in nature, outside. This makes it harder for our bodies to regulate sleep time and other bodily functions like hunger.

Americans have been funding a *Sleep Better Now!* industry to the tune of billions of dollars for decades because we are looking for quick answers to our poor nights of sleep. We forget that having one or two nights of poor sleep monthly is normal. We expect to have excellent sleep night after night and lose sight of sleep being a drive, not a talent. Instead of working on it to strengthen our sleep habits, we try adding in new things (Supplements! Pillows! Socks! Lamps!) to make sleep "easier."

The technology now exists to do things we never dreamed possible. I know every generation has been able to say this for many decades, but today, our technology has evolved in ways we couldn't have anticipated. We have social media and games (small and large) that can connect us immediately and for as long as we like to software that instantly responds to our input and provides us with colorful, exciting, and horrifying images that are specifically designed to keep our brains interested and invested in staying. From cat videos to *Call of Duty*, we have never had technology better designed to trick our brains into feeling active and alert while we are essentially sitting still.

### Catching a Wave or the Perfect Cookie Recipe

And then there is the effort to create perfect sleep.

When I meet new clients with sleep problems, the first several minutes of our conversations often consist of them explaining to me how worried they are that their process of getting to sleep has failed them. Usually the problem starts innocently enough—they have a few bad nights of sleep, often due to an identifiable cause (work or home stress, illness or injury, in short: life happens), and they add something to their bedtime routine to make it more likely that they will have a better night of sleep. Let's say they start with a new pillow. It seems to help a bit. Great! Why not add something else? Surely, it can get better. Maybe a white noise machine; maybe some fancy sheets. Maybe a supplement that your neighbor's cousin swears helps her sleep soundly night after night.

Megan is a new client and is telling me about her recent efforts to improve her sleep: She bought a new pillow, then a white noise machine, then she started taking melatonin, then she read about tart cherry juice and added that to her routine, then blue-blocker glasses after sundown, then yoga Nidra an hour before bed and chamomile tea after yoga Nidra, then a warm shower (not too hot, not too cold), and so on, and so on. Megan ends this description with exasperation: "I'm doing all of these things right; so why is my sleep still so bad?"

I call this seeking the "perfect cookie recipe." Megan is focused on several activities and has bought several products that she has come to rely on to sleep. Notice that several of the items Megan is using are generally positive or helpful for sleep; none of them is wrong if used correctly. The problem becomes the effort and the expectation that these items or activities, when performed properly or when lined up in just the right order and timed correctly, will always produce a great night of sleep. There is no perfect recipe for falling and staying asleep every night for every person. With cookies, even if you maintain strict ingredients and mixing, the difference in weather can change the taste of the cookie. With sleep, I'll go out on a limb and say that there is not a perfect set of activities for any one person that will create perfect sleep every night. Humans, and our messy lives, aren't that simple. The good news is that sleep is a drive. Sleep is resilient to your efforts and will come eventually, even if the effort you make toward sleep is enough to keep you awake longer. Let's get into that idea.

You may be an expert cookie baker. Being an expert at anything takes a lot of effort and intention. Unfortunately for you, no matter how well you make cookies most of the time, it only takes some humidity, a very cold kitchen, or some slightly older eggs for them to taste different from the last "perfect" batch. Even if you slept "exactly like last night," and everything worked so well you "slept for eight hours," things can change outside of your control and impact your sleep: The weather changes, someone coughs, or the door opens, and your cookies are different. Stress and illness are two common disturbances that can disrupt sleep. But common things like dehydration, temperature changes (outside and inside of your sleep environment), nutrition, exercise, travel, and so on can disrupt just as much or more.

My point here is not that you need to overcome all the things that can disrupt your sleep and always sleep perfectly. My point is the opposite of that. I want you to think of your sleep as resilient. Remember, at the end of the day, sleep is a drive like hunger and thirst; your body will get the sleep it needs. Cookies baked in high humidity or with ingredients that weren't perfectly fresh are still tasty.

### Surfing with Megan

When I worked with Megan and her list of items that she used in pursuit of excellent sleep, our first step was to work on a metaphor. Megan understood the "cookie recipe" issue, but she asked, "If I'm not curating my own sleep recipe, then what am I supposed to focus on while I'm getting ready for bed?"

I told Megan to think of getting ready for bed like getting ready to go surfing. Surfing isn't an activity you can do the same way every time, and there are many aspects you can't control—especially the waves. Megan's new goal was to get herself in the right place (her comfortable bed), at the right time (when she feels sleepy), and in the right frame of mind (appreciating her opportunity for calm recovery) and then to wait for the sleep wave to arrive. Just like surfing, if you miss the first wave, another one will arrive soon enough.

Sleep will always be different on different nights and different for different people. Humans don't have perfect sleep night after night, month after month. Most of us who sleep well have a poor night one or two times every month. However, there are ways to improve your sleep and make it resistant to ongoing sleep difficulties. You can learn to let go of the pressure to sleep well, learn how to help your body regulate wake and sleep time, and then get out of its way so that it can do the job it was built to do.

Megan loved the surfing metaphor, and she really got into it, even buying some sea glass to keep on her bedside table as a reminder. She kept her pillow, would drink tart cherry juice when she wanted to, and eased up on all her effort to get the perfect night of sleep. It wasn't long before her sleep was more relaxing, and her worry about how her night was going changed into a calmness about bedtime being her "surfing zen zone."

She emailed me months after we finished our work and said that she mentioned the "surfing the waves of sleep" idea to a friend, and her friend couldn't get it. "I think she's afraid of surfing and the ocean in general," she wrote. Metaphors are like this—they don't work for everyone.

I wrote her back, "Tell your friend another way to think about getting ready for sleep is like when you visit a friend who has a cat that you want to pet. The harder you try to pet the cat, the less successful you are going to be. But if you put yourself in the right frame of mind (calm, relaxed) and in the right place (sitting quietly, not staring at the cat), it won't be long before the cat is seeking you out." Megan wrote me a week later to say her friend loved that metaphor and was using it as her imagery before bed every night.

Here's the tricky part of what we are doing here: Aspects of this book may feel like I'm encouraging you to create your own cookie recipe—do them right to make certain you will sleep perfectly. That's a misunderstanding of my efforts. You will notice me encouraging you to learn new strategies you can incorporate, and once they are routine, to stop thinking about them, so sleep can become less intentional and more automatic. I want this to be a new solid structure for sleep: not the perfect cookie recipe but more like tips on how to prepare yourself to calmly surf the waves of sleep.

In the next section, I will help you understand how your body and brain are built to create sleepiness, to allow for some poor nights of sleep and still be healthy, and to get the sleep that you need. I'm not here to scare you about your sleep, and I won't make you fearful about what product you are missing out on and need to buy immediately. That's not your problem; I'm almost certain. I'll start with some top-level sleep tips in this section, and then in the third section, I'll wrap those tips into a package called the *Camping Sleep Reset* that brings all the ideas and tips together.

CHAPTER 2

# WHAT IS SLEEP AND HOW MUCH DO I NEED?

The science of sleep began with Nathaniel Kleitman and William Dement in Chicago in 1957, when they noticed and coined the term *rapid eye movement* for what happens during the dreaming stage of sleep.[17] Over the seventy years since then, so much has been learned about what sleep is, what it does for our bodies and minds, and how it misfires at times.

If you want to dive deeper into the details of sleep science, I have suggestions at the end of this book. (There are so many excellent books, lectures, and YouTube channels where sleep is described in detail.) But for my purposes here, I want you to know a few key things. First, sleep is vital to your health and your mental health. Poor sleep leads to a weakened immune system, difficulty managing emotions, irritability, lowered creativity, and an increase in thoughts of suicide. Chronic sleep problems lasting decades appear to contribute to other severe health issues like heart disease, stroke, and dementia. It's difficult to pinpoint causes, but the sleep scientists are getting closer to doing so all the time.

When I talk to groups about sleep, I sometimes narrow it down to three things that sleep does that everyone I've met cares about. First, sleep helps us stay healthy. When I suffered from sleep apnea as a teenager, I caught every cold, flu, and virus that went around. Once my nasal blockage was fixed, I stopped catching all those colds.

Second, sleep makes us more attractive. The research John Axelsson[18] and Tim Sundelin[19] and their team completed at Stolkhom University in 2010 and again in 2017 used dozens of volunteers' photos after getting plenty of sleep and then deprived the same people of sleep for two days and took photos again. The photos were controlled for lighting, angles, and everything that could make them look different. The photos were shown to vast groups of people who were asked to rate the attractiveness of each participant. Guess what? When well rested, the same person was rated as more attractive than when sleep deprived.

Third, sleep helps us maintain a healthy weight. There are many factors that go into this, but one that you haven't heard is how our eating hormones are affected by sleep. Ghrelin and leptin are the hormones our bodies use to let us know when we are hungry or full, respectively. When we are sleep-deprived, these hormones are impacted. Delaney Gresser explains that without enough sleep, ghrelin goes into overdrive and encourages us to eat more. One hypothesis I have is that this may happen because our brains interpret limited sleep as a symptom of danger—and eating more is a protection from starvation in uncertain circumstances. Meanwhile, leptin levels are reduced without sufficient sleep, making our bodies unclear when we are full.[20]

Why care about sleep? Because sleep holds our bodies together physically and emotionally. When you do it well most of the time, you will be healthier, more attractive, and have an easier time maintaining a healthy weight.

## WHAT HAPPENS AT NIGHT?

I'm going to keep this brief, but I want you to know a few things about your sleep and your sleep stages. The most important thing to know about your sleep stages and cycles of sleep is that your body knows what it is doing. You don't have to do anything for your sleep cycles and sleep stages to work properly—your brain and body will do that for you. Spoiler alert: Despite what you may have heard, there is variability from night to night between how much time a healthy sleeper spends in different sleep stages based on several factors.

### Cycles

Over the course of a night of sleep, you will experience a few sleep cycles. Each cycle consists of the four major sleep stages: stage 1, stage 2, deep sleep, and REM sleep. Each cycle of sleep lasts over an hour, and the longer you sleep in a night, the longer the cycles tend to last, up to as much as two hours.

Let me open your eyes a little further: Each sleep cycle is different from the one before it. The first cycle of the night will have the longest period of deep sleep, and each cycle after that will have a shorter stage of deep sleep than the one prior. On the other hand, the first cycle of the night will have the shortest REM stage of the night, and each cycle after that will have a longer stage of REM sleep than the one prior. This complex balance of longer and shorter stages is also different each night for each person based on several things, like exercise, distress, nutrition, hydration, health, and alcohol.

**Stage 1** sleep is the lightest stage. This is a transitional stage from being awake to being asleep. For most of us, most of the time, this is a very brief stage of sleep, lasting just several minutes. On the other hand, if you are under a great deal of distress and you have been lying in bed "awake for hours" but can't account for what you've been doing all that time, it's likely because you were lapsing in and out of stage 1 sleep and wakefulness. That's not good sleep.

If I woke you from stage 1, you would tell me you weren't asleep; you were just resting quietly. It is sleep—but it doesn't feel like sleep because you are in the transition from being awake to being asleep.

**Stage 2** sleep is pure light sleep. During the night, you'll spend most of your time in stage 2 sleep. This is a transition period from wakefulness, just a bit deeper than stage 1. This stage is essential to getting good sleep because you use stage 2 to get to the next stages.

If I woke you from stage 2, it wouldn't be hard—you'd be alert relatively quickly, but you would also be clear that you had been asleep.

**Deep sleep** is the stage where your body makes its recovery. During deep sleep your immune system gets its biggest boost of the twenty-four-hour cycle. When you do heavy physical labor or exercise or when you are ill or injured, your body and brain add more time to your deep sleep stage for additional recovery. A simple way to think of deep sleep is as a physical recovery period. Much more than that happens here, but it's a good shorthand.

If I woke you from deep sleep, it would be hard—your brain and body are essentially in a power-down mode, and it takes a while for you to restart. Waking someone from deep sleep is challenging—they seem disoriented and confused.

**REM sleep** is just what you think it is, and so much more. REM sleep is dream sleep. While we sometimes have brief dreams in other stages of sleep, nearly all the dreams we have are in REM sleep. Dreaming is our brain's way of reprocessing our challenging or difficult experiences, problems you are trying to work out but especially emotionally upsetting experiences. A simple way to think of REM sleep is as a mental and emotional recovery period.

If I woke you from REM sleep, you would remember that you were dreaming and would feel mentally alert, especially compared to waking from other stages. While your brain is very active, your body is immobilized during REM due to a natural spinal block so that you don't act out those dreams you are having. If woken from REM, your brain will take several long seconds or up to a minute or two to allow your body to arrive at functional. If you've ever experienced sleep paralysis (being unable to move upon waking for a minute or so), you have woken from REM so quickly that the spinal block hasn't been removed yet. This is rare, but it happens to most people once in a while.

## Wearables and Orthosomnia

Maybe you have an Apple Watch, a Fitbit, a Garmin, a Whoop band, an Oura ring, or a mattress or pillow that "measures" your sleep and gives you a score and an update each morning on how you slept. These wearables have some amazing features that have alerted millions of people to sleep patterns suggestive of obstructive sleep apnea or other problems. It's great when technology improves things and assists in getting tested and treated for sleep disorders! It's a win!

On the other hand, like anything one pays too much attention to, sleep tracking can be a slippery slope into paying so much attention to sleep data that a person develops a hyperfocus on sleep that leads to insomnia.

In the world of eating disorders, there is a proposed diagnosis called orthorexia. People suffering from orthorexia spend so much time and effort eating healthily that they develop secondary problems like anxiety, isolation, and an inability to eat in a natural, intuitive way. Ortho*somnia* is the concept of obsessively focusing on sleep data from sleep trackers—so much so that sleep is negatively impacted.

I wear sleep trackers myself, but I maintain a healthy relationship with them by keeping a few things in mind:

- If it feels like I'm getting overwhelmed by the data, I can always turn it off. I slept without a wearable for most of my life and had no problems.
- Wearables measure things that are related to sleep—heart rate, movement, blood oxygenation, and so on. What is missing from that list? Brain waves. The only way to accurately track sleep staging is via brain waves. Apple, Garmin, Oura, Whoop, Fitbit and the rest of the trackers are taking their best guess at how much time you spend in each sleep stage based on several factors but not your brain waves. They are pretty accurate, but they are often wrong.
- My sleep is personal to me and my life. Being told by an algorithm that I only had three minutes of deep sleep last night, or that my recovery score was a 5 out of 100, means something was off—but I'm going to trust how I feel today much more than I'm going to trust my watch.

There is so much more to know about sleep cycles and stages, but this is what you need to know for our work here. Later, I'll tell you about how the sleep stages are like Disney World and how to maximize your experience in the park.

## How Much Sleep Do I Need?

This is probably the most asked question I get when I tell people what I do on a plane or while sitting in a jury duty room. Everyone knows the answer, right? It's eight. Isn't it? Well, yes and no, and not really.

First, let's address the idea of "sleep need." What a person *wants* and what they *need* are often very, very different. When you go out to dinner, you may want a hot bowl of ramen with a beautiful side of steamed dumplings. But what you need to survive are enough calories and nutrition for your body to get through your day. While you want the ramen and dumplings, you could eat rice and beans for most meals during the week and have what you *need* to survive.

The amount of sleep you need to survive is much less than eight hours per night. But that won't last long. You can survive on only a little sleep for a while, but diminished sleep will take a toll on you—especially your immune system and your mental health. The longer you go with diminished sleep, the worse your body will operate in nearly every way.

But that's not what you meant when you asked the question, was it? What you meant was "How much sleep should I be getting most nights?" That's an even better question. But if you thought I'd have a simple answer, prepare to be disappointed. That said, you may learn something, so buckle in.

If I'm talking to a group of one thousand people, and I need a quick answer that's going to be accurate for the most people, then yes, the answer is about seven and a half hours. Because that's a good general answer for a large group of people. Seven and a half hours for most people is plenty of sleep and will allow them to operate at their best. But it's just you reading this book, not the masses, and to get more accurate information, I need to know more about you.

The first thing I need to know is your age. According to the National Sleep Foundation, newborns and infants need the most sleep, as much as 19 hours per day, but they rarely ask me for sleep advice.[21] Toddlers and preschool-aged kids are recommended to get 10–14 hours per night. Kids in grade school through the age of thirteen are recommended to get 9–11 hours per night. If you are a parent and reading this, you should pat yourself on the back if your kids are getting enough sleep. If you feel surprised kids need so much sleep, talk to your pediatrician or find one of the great books out there about kids and sleep from people like Jodi Mindell or Lisa Meltzer. Two of the greatest things you can teach your children to support their physical health, mental health, and life skills are to have good boundaries and respect for sleep. Just reading this book in front of them is a step in the right direction. Helping them take their own sleep seriously is even more important. Great research from Michelle Short and Mary Carskadon back in 2011 showed that adults who grew up with good sleep boundaries (set by parents), like when to be in bed and having phones outside of bedrooms, are much healthier and more successful adults.[22] Imagine helping your kids live healthier lives just by keeping a consistent bedtime and phone usage boundaries. It's easier than it sounds, and it's not expensive or complicated.

If you're not a kid but an adult, then the answer to how much sleep you need is nuanced. There are two reliable sources that seem to disagree on this. The National Sleep Foundation recommends 7–9 hours for adults[23] but acknowledges that it may be appropriate for some adults to get as little as 6 hours and others as much as 11 hours. Research from Daniel Kripke, a leader in the field of sleep medicine, looked at the sleep experiences of over one million people and found that the optimal sleep range is 6.5–7.4 hours.[24]

The two sources give similar recommendations but for different reasons. The National Sleep Foundation wants you to know that sleep needs vary widely. Kripke and the field of sleep medicine want you to know that most people do well to get between 6.5 and 7.5 hours per night of sleep. And those same people may need even more or even less some days, depending on their activities and stress level. Older adults sleep a little bit less than younger adults, but not by much.

Think of 7.5 hours as a good average. There are more than 8 billion people in the world, and most of them are adults. Let's say there are 6 billion adults. If they all got 7.5 hours of sleep most nights, most of them would function at their best.

Nearly every adult is at their best when they are getting more than 7 hours of sleep per night. But those who think they are doing great with 5 hours are unlikely to be convinced that they aren't doing great with less. Like driving, it may be apparent to everyone around them through their irritability, drowsiness, and general grumpiness, but an unfortunate part of the experience of being chronically tired is rigidity: less openness to ideas or constructive feedback about their fatigue and sleep.

And not coincidentally, a sleep-deprived person is also an impaired driver. The Governor's Highway Safety Panel created a graphic to show how impaired a driver is based on their hours of sleep deprivation

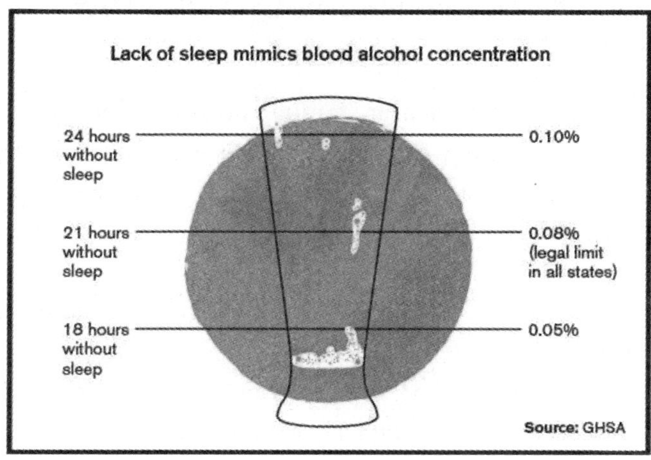


## Track your Energy and Mood for Four Weeks

Giving up on the idea that you are one of the special people who need less sleep than 99% of adults could help you feel better and live healthier. Don't believe me? Try it out for four weeks by experimenting on yourself—what do you have to lose? Use the table below to track your health and happiness, as well as your sleep, for two weeks just the way you are. Change nothing but monitor how you sleep, how you feel each day, and your happiness levels. For the next two weeks, dedicate eight hours per night to sleep. You probably won't sleep all eight hours every night because sleep needs change a bit from day to day (see the next section) but make eight hours of sleep time a daily priority. See how your life changes. And check in with those around you—your family members, friends, and colleagues. Ask at least one of them what they think about your mood and energy level once a week. Their opinion matters to you, right? So ask!

## WHY DO MY SLEEP NEEDS CHANGE DAY TO DAY?

Let me help make this clearer. Jamila is training for a marathon. Wednesday is a light day of training for her when she does yoga for forty minutes in her apartment, where she can control the temperature to be about 72 degrees with little humidity. She spends the rest of her day in an air-conditioned office sitting down.

On a day like this, Jamila will drink between four and six large glasses of water.

On Saturday, Jamila will run fourteen miles when it's 80 degrees outside and moderate humidity. That run will take her just less than two hours because Jamila is a fantastic runner.

When Jamila drinks four to six large glasses of water on Saturday, will she be hydrated for the day? Of course not. She may need twelve glasses of water today to keep hydrated after such a demanding workout in the heat and some humidity.

People don't wonder why they are thirstier on hot days when they are exercising a lot than on cool days when they are sitting still. People

| Day | Time To Bed | Minutes to Fall Asleep | Minutes Awake Overnight | Time Out of Bed | Total Sleep Time | Energy Level (1/Low-10/High) | Mood (1/Low-10/High) | Partner/ Friend Rates my Mood (1/Low-10/High) |
|---|---|---|---|---|---|---|---|---|
| Example | 11:30 pm | 15 min | 30 min | 6:15am | 6 h 0 min | 5 | 6 | 5 |
| 1 | | | | | | | | |
| 2 | | | | | | | | |
| 3 | | | | | | | | |
| 4 | | | | | | | | |
| 5 | | | | | | | | |
| 6 | | | | | | | | |
| 7 | | | | | | | | |
| 8 | | | | | | | | |
| 9 | | | | | | | | |
| 10 | | | | | | | | |
| 11 | | | | | | | | |
| 12 | | | | | | | | |
| 13 | | | | | | | | |
| 14 | | | | | | | | |

| Prioritizing 8 Hours of Sleep | Time to Bed | Minutes to Fall Asleep | Minutes Awake Overnight | Time Out of Bed | Total Sleep Time | Energy Level (1/Low-10/High) | Mood (1/Low-10/High) | Partner/ Friend Rates my Mood (1/Low-10/High) |
|---|---|---|---|---|---|---|---|---|
| 15 | | | | | | | | |
| 16 | | | | | | | | |
| 17 | | | | | | | | |
| 18 | | | | | | | | |
| 19 | | | | | | | | |
| 20 | | | | | | | | |
| 21 | | | | | | | | |
| 22 | | | | | | | | |
| 23 | | | | | | | | |
| 24 | | | | | | | | |
| 25 | | | | | | | | |
| 26 | | | | | | | | |
| 27 | | | | | | | | |
| 28 | | | | | | | | |

just understand that they need more hydration when they are doing more.

Sleep is the same, just less obvious. Both sleep and thirst are human drives: You need them to survive. So, when you demand more from your body, the drive for these things will increase. Simple, right?

## HOW DO I DETERMINE HOW MANY HOURS OF SLEEP I NEED TO FUNCTION AT MY BEST?

If you've stuck with me long enough to read through the previous section, you probably want to know if it's possible to determine how much sleep your body needs to function at its best. There's good news and bad news . . .

Good news: The answer is yes, and the bonus answer—it's free!

Bad news: To do this well, you need to have flexibility in your schedule for ten days to two weeks. Not everyone can take two weeks of vacation or roll into work at whatever time they happen to wake up for a couple of weeks. Whether you are one of the lucky people who can or not, there are techniques to take away from this that can help guide you to what your body wants.

I start this process with the assumption that you struggle with feeling like you get enough sleep. If you have a job, are a full-time student, or are a member of the military, it's a good guess. If you happen to be well rested, this will be a quicker process for you.

In a nutshell, while you can never make up for the lost sleep you missed, you will sleep off as much of your sleep debt as possible in about a week's worth of time. That means that once you've arrived at the "caught up on sleep" mark, your body only needs to sleep the next night as much as it needs to get you through your day at a high level of functioning—it no longer needs to spend time trying to catch up on lost sleep. Remember that your brain and your body have multiple internal systems designed to know how much sleep you need to function at your best. This process of learning how much sleep you need relies on those internal systems to do their job.

Your job is to create a consistent block of time at night for your body to sleep as much as it wants. You need to plan on doing this for two weeks. The more well rested you are when you begin, the less time this will take—but for most of us, ten days to two weeks is a good estimate.

Committing to the time for sleep can be the hardest part. It's easy to commit to sleeping as much as you want on a weekend, or after a tough day or two at work. But for this plan to work, you need to commit to and follow through with allowing yourself to sleep as much as you can for two weeks. For most people, this means sleeping without your alarm and getting up when you wake up. For some people, it means getting to bed when sleepy—not pushing past sleepiness for another episode of *The Good Place* or to check email again.

This is hard because most of us have obligations in the morning and some of us in the evening, and others have both. Do you have children in the house? Then you have both. Do you have someone who relies on you for their care? A pet or a loved one with special needs? Then you have obligations that make this challenging.

Many of the people I have helped through this process have done so during a vacation or a break. College students have built-in breaks between semesters and often can use two weeks of them for this. Older adults without kids or pets do well with these instructions because most of their obligations are their own.

Figure out when this will work for you. Maybe use the last three days of your work week to sleep before starting a week of vacation where you can follow through each night for a total of ten nights. That's great!

If it doesn't work for you and your lifestyle, hang on to the idea for a time when it might.

*Caveat: If you are suffering from an untreated sleep disorder, a chronic health problem, or heavy substance use, this will not work for you. If you try this for a solid two weeks and never notice a reduction in sleep amount, you should consider talking to your doctor about what is causing your heavy sleep need.*

Here are the steps for determining how much sleep you need:

**1. Track your sleep before and during this process. Sleep tracking is how you measure how much sleep you need—It's essential! Note the following:**

- What time did you go to bed?
- What time did you wake up?
- How much time were you not sleeping during the time you set aside to sleep?
- And most importantly, how much sleep did you get last night?

**2. Commit to the process. When it's time, set aside at least ten days and probably about fourteen nights where you can sleep as much as your body wants.**

**3. Avoid common disruptors—no naps, no alcohol, and no cannabis while you are working on this. And no caffeine after noon.**

**4. Track your daily well-being. At the end of each day, note how you felt throughout your waking hours. How was your energy? How was your mood?**

### Ben's Sleeping Experiment

Ben was a college student and generally healthy. He didn't drink much or smoke at all, and he was frustrated because he often spent his weekends catching up on the lost sleep from the week. During the week he would sleep about six hours per night, and then on Friday and Saturday night he would catch up by sleeping ten to twelve hours per night.

We worked on his time management and his depressed mood in therapy. Then he asked if I could help him determine how much sleep he should prioritize during the week. He wanted to enjoy his weekends rather than sleeping twenty-two hours between Friday night and Sunday morning.

He committed to the two weeks after finals to be his experiment time. He was returning to work for the summer but was approved to take afternoon or evening shifts for those first two weeks.

The first three nights he slept between ten and twelve hours, which is exactly what he expected based on previous experience. It was night five when Ben emailed me to say he was worried. He still got nine hours of sleep that night and thought he might be learning that his body wanted him to live with nine hours per night for the rest of his life. I encouraged him to pace himself and not make any conclusions until he was done. The experiment had only just started. He returned to the process feeling more hopeful.

I met with him again after the ninth night, and here's what we looked at together:

| Day | Time to Bed | Minutes to Fall Asleep | Minutes Awake Overnight | Time Out of Bed | Total Sleep Time | Energy Level (1/Low-10/ High) | Mood (1/Low-10/High) |
|---|---|---|---|---|---|---|---|
| 1 Sun-Mon morning | 12:15 am | 15 min | 5 min | 11:55 am | 11h 25min | 5 | 3 |
| 2 Mon-Tue morning | 12:00 am | 20 min | 15 min | 11:50 am | 11h 15min | 5 | 4 |
| 3 Tue-Wed morning | 11:45 pm | 20 min | 5 min | 10:15 am | 10h 5min | 6 | 4 |
| 4 Wed-Thurs morning | 12:00 am | 15 min | 0 min | 10:00 am | 9h 45min | 5 | 4 |
| 5 Thurs-Fri morning | 11:45 pm | 20 min | 10 min | 9:10 am | 8h 55min | 6 | 5 |
| 6 Fri-Sat morning | 12:00 am | 15 min | 0 min | 9:00 am | 8h 45min | 6 | 7 |
| 7 Sat-Sun morning | 12:15 am | 10 min | 15 min | 7:30 am | 7h 5min | 5 | 6 |
| 8 Sun-Mon morning | 11:45 pm | 5 min | 10 min | 9:15 am | 9h 00min | 7 | 7 |
| 9 Mon-Tue morning | 12:30 am | 15 min | 0 min | 8:00 am | 7h 45min | 7 | 8 |

The first few nights, there was a large amount of sleep debt to pay off, and Ben did it. He slept like he did most of his weekends during college—over eleven hours per night. There were no other nights when he was able to sleep more than eleven hours, even though he was allowing as much sleep as his body would use. There were no alarms set, no place to be until more than sixteen hours after he went to bed.

As the sleep debt slowly declined, Ben also started experiencing more energy during the day and a better mood. These scores are subjective, meaning Ben was scoring his own energy and mood. But to be fair, who cares more about Ben's energy and mood than Ben?

As the nights went on and Ben was carrying less sleep debt, he slept less because his body was more rested. After Ben completed two full weeks of sleeping as late as his body would allow, here is what he saw:

| Day | Total Sleep Time | Energy Level (1/Low- 10/High) | Mood (1/Low- 10/High) |
|---|---|---|---|
| 1 Sun-Mon morning | 11h 25min | 5 | 3 |
| 2 Mon-Tue morning | 11h 15min | 5 | 4 |
| 3 Tue-Wed morning | 10h 5min | 6 | 4 |
| 4 Wed-Thurs morning | 9h 45min | 5 | 4 |
| 5 Thurs-Fri morning | 8h 55min | 6 | 5 |
| 6 Fri-Sat morning | 8h 45min | 6 | 7 |
| 7 Sat-Sun morning | 7h 5min | 5 | 6 |
| 8 Sun-Mon morning | 9h 00min | 7 | 7 |
| 9 Mon-Tue morning | 7h 45min | 7 | 8 |
| 10 Tue-Wed morning | 7h 50min | 8 | 8 |
| 11 Wed-Thur morning | 7h 25min | 7 | 8 |
| 12 Thur-Fri morning | 7h 45min | 7 | 7 |
| 13 Fri-Sat morning | 7h 5min | 9 | 8 |
| 14 Sat-Sun morning | 7h 30min | 9 | 9 |
| 15 Sun-Mon morning | 7h 20min | 8 | 7 |

Ben was excited to tell me that he hadn't felt like this since he was a kid. He felt consistent energy throughout the day. He knew it was about time to go to bed when he was feeling sleepy—not just when it was time for bed—and he felt healthy. His friends were asking him what was different about him or what he was taking to make him seem so different. The answer was sleep and enough of it.

Ben was also pleased to tell me that it became clear that he needs about 7 hours and 20 minutes to 7 hours and 45 minutes of sleep nightly, based on his day. When he is well rested and has a challenging day, he needs a bit more; when his day is milder, he needs a bit less. He was amazed at how obvious this seemed in hindsight.

I stressed to him that when he catches a cold, has a very stressful day, or exercises more intensely, he will likely need more sleep. But the benefit of knowing how much sleep he needs is that Ben can plan to get about 7 hours and 30 minutes of sleep most of the time, and then when he has a difficult day, he can plan to sleep a bit more.

This is a much better strategy than sleeping 6 hours per night for five nights and then trying to catch up on the 7 hours and 30 minutes of sleep debt over the weekend. Ben learned that he was short-changing himself one whole night of sleep per week during the weeknights and then short-changing his weekend "fun time" by sleeping an extra 7 hours, so he could return to equilibrium.

I saw Ben again on campus about a year later and asked him how it was going. He told me that he doesn't always sleep 7 hours and 30 minutes every night, but he rarely sleeps as little as 6 hours because he can feel the deficit it puts him in. And he knows that if he must have a shorter night of sleep, or if he has a very stressful day, he will plan to get a bit more sleep than usual to get back on track.

All in all, he said, he is more regular with his sleep. He hovers closer to 7 hours and 30 minutes every night. On weekends he will get something more like 8 hours and 30 minutes because it feels good, but he also knows not to oversleep on weekends because it can wreck his

Sunday night—making it harder to fall asleep and wake up on Monday morning. He was on a new track and glad he tried the sleep challenge to know what he needed.

## My Bedpartner Snores. Should I Send Them to See You?

One of the reasons that the experiment above could fail for millions of people is obstructive sleep apnea (OSA). If you tried it for several days and your hours of sleep never dropped, you may be dealing with a sleep disorder like OSA. It could also be a problem with your iron or your thyroid or be related to another health or sleep problem. But if you are a snorer, OSA is the first thing to investigate with your doctor.

Snoring is one of the most easily recognizable signs of OSA. According to the American Academy of Sleep Medicine, approximately 30 million Americans are estimated to have obstructive sleep apnea, yet only 6 million have received a formal diagnosis—which suggests that 80% of cases remain undiagnosed. Untreated OSA correlates highly with heart attacks, strokes, and car accidents (people with OSA often fall asleep while driving due to chronic daytime sleepiness).[25]

While snoring is the symptom most people recognize as related to OSA, snoring doesn't always mean one has OSA. In fact, most adults snore a bit, especially while sleeping on their backs.

If your child snores—that's a different story. Most children do not snore, and a child who snores is likely dealing with an airway issue like the one I dealt with growing up. Take your child to their pediatrician and tell the doctor that you are concerned they may have apnea due to their snoring. Children often hide fatigue well, but the ramifications of growing up with an airway that is chronically blocked during sleep can also be severe.

Snoring means that there is difficulty breathing—the airway isn't fully open, which makes the snore happen. The louder the snore, the more likely OSA is present. If someone can hear you snoring through the door or down the hall, you are a loud snorer, and I would recommend you speak with your physician about it.

On the other hand, some people who do not snore at all are also suffering from OSA. So let's not get hung up on snoring.

When I hear a question like this from a client or audience member, my next question is whether they wake up choking or gasping for breath. This is a much stronger indicator of OSA than snoring. The next question is how tired they feel during the day. OSA is consistently disruptive to sleep; therefore, people with OSA remain exhausted after spending long hours sleeping.

Other indicators for OSA include your neck size, your weight (having obesity or being overweight), and your airway structure (having a narrow airway and a thick, soft palate). Additional risk factors include smoking, drinking alcohol regularly, sedative use, and being menopausal or postmenopausal. Medical conditions such as heart disease, stroke, diabetes, hypertension, nasal congestion, and thyroid disorder can also increase your risk for OSA. Research from Tina Ghavami[26] and her team shows that the older we get, the higher the likelihood of having OSA. David Dancey[27] and his team, and many others in the decades since, found that while OSA is more common in men, upon reaching menopause, women quickly catch up, unfortunately. Multiple studies have shown that medications like benzodiazepines and opioids can worsen symptoms of OSA and make it more problematic.[28]

Bottom line—if these risk factors sound like you, you should be talking to your primary care physician about the likelihood of having OSA, even if you've been tested before. I have had clients tell me that they snore and were tested for OSA, and it was found to be minor or not an issue. That's great news but remember that OSA is a progressive disorder for most people, meaning just because your OSA was minor five or ten years ago does not mean it has remained stable. Unless you have lost a lot of weight since your test, your OSA will naturally worsen as you age. If you are experiencing these symptoms, talk to your primary care physician even if you had a negative test for OSA in the past.

## CAN I REPAY MY SLEEP DEBT? IS IT EVEN A REAL THING?

I love getting this question because I know the person asking it has either been listening closely or has already given this some thought.

This answer is more nuanced than most people are excited to hear. To explain the answer, I remind people of all the ways sleep helps our bodies. It boosts our immune systems, manages our emotional life and makes us feel more upbeat, helps us be more creative, promotes more coordination in our movements (like driving a car), and helps us remember things better and connect new information with older information. Sounds familiar, right?

Let me use an example to make this abundantly clear. Let's say my buddy Steve underslept by two hours the whole work week, and by Friday night, he accrued almost eight hours of sleep debt. Then he tried to catch up over the weekend, sleeping almost ten hours on Friday night and over ten hours on Saturday night. By Sunday morning he still had three hours and forty minutes of sleep debt remaining from his week. Even if he were able to sleep an additional eight hours over the weekend (beyond his standard need for nightly sleep), he could never get back the limited functioning he lived with during that week—that ship has sailed.

### Steve's Week Developing Sleep Debt and Using the Weekend to "Sleep It Off"

| Day | Time to Bed | Minutes to Fall Asleep | Minutes Awake Overnight | Time Out of Bed | Total Sleep Time | Accumulated Sleep Debt |
|---|---|---|---|---|---|---|
| 1 Sun-Mon morning | 11:30 pm | 15 min | 5 min | 6:50 am | 6h 0min | -2 hours |
| 2 Mon-Tue morning | 12:00 am | 20 min | 15 min | 7:00 am | 6h 25min | -3h35min |
| 3 Tue-Wed morning | 11:30 pm | 10 min | 5 min | 6:45 am | 7h 0min | 4h 35min |
| 4 Wed-Thurs morning | 1:00 am | 5 min | 0 min | 6:45 am | 5h 40min | 6h 55min |
| 5 Thurs-Fri morning | 11:45 pm | 10 min | 15 min | 7:10 am | 7h 0min | 7h 55min |
| 6 Fri-Sat morning | 12:00 am | 15 min | 0 min | 10:00 am | 9h 45min | 6h 10min |
| 7 Sat-Sun morning | 11:30 pm | 10 min | 20 min | 10:30 am | 10h 30min | 3h 40min |

On Wednesday, Steve had already accrued four and a half hours of sleep debt, lowering his immune system's ability a bit. That was the day he had a meeting with his coworker John, who didn't know it yet but was about to come down with a nasty cold. They were in the same room talking for an hour and shared a few jokes, so John spewed cold virus all around the room after each joke. C'mon, John. That's gross.

On Thursday, Steve had nearly seven hours of sleep debt, slowing his reaction time from its optimum, when he is fully rested. That was the day he had a fender bender with the car in front of him because he didn't stop quickly enough at a red light.

On Friday, Steve bumped into that neighbor he met once and who borrowed the pan Steve likes to cook his enchiladas in. At this point, he had nearly eight hours of sleep debt accrued, and his mind wasn't as sharp as it is when he is well rested. He really wants that pan back, but he couldn't come up with the neighbor's name in the fifteen seconds they saw one another and spent the exchange trying to come up with her name rather than ask about the pan. (It's Erica.)

So, did sleeping in on Saturday and getting extra hours of sleep pay off Steve's sleep debt? Well, it helped his body recover from some of its losses. But Steve can't go back in time to remember Erica's name and get the pan back, have better reaction time to avoid the fender bender, or have a stronger immune system to fight off John's cold. That opportunity has passed.

It's not all doom and gloom, though. "Catching up on sleep" is a real thing. While what's done is done, you still make gains when you get recovery sleep beyond your standard need. In fact, you can also look at sleep debt as a temporary change in your sleep need.

Let's say Steve goes through his weekend and gets an extra four hours and fifteen minutes of sleep beyond his standard sleep need of eight hours. If he times his waking well, he will start the week strong. He will have a replenished immune system and a sharp memory that is ready for new ideas and information. Whether he was showing symptoms from John's cold on Friday or not, he is likely fighting it off as effectively as he can after two extra sleep nights. And when he sees Erica again at the store on Sunday night, he will remember her name and get his pan back. Life is good.

Bottom line: Recovering sleep debt is not an "hour extra for every hour lost" equation. Take my experience, for example. Because of my severely deviated septum, I grew up with an ongoing sleep debt for my entire childhood. I could sleep in on weekends, but I could never get the chance to catch up on my massive sleep debt—it was just gone. I did pay for it nearly every day: I caught all the colds and flus that came through school, I had social challenges, and I struggled with things like driving without falling asleep. That was my life as someone with a septum-induced obstructive sleep apnea.

For those of you who aren't dealing with a sleep disorder, I like to provide the guidance that you can make up for about the last three nights of sleep debt. The science around this is hotly debated, but this is my personal belief based on my experience and that of those I've worked with. Beyond that, it's more important to focus on tonight and living well. This is a longer, usually unwanted, answer to the question "Why do I feel tired all day after I've slept in?" The answer is that you are feeling the effects of the previous three nights today. You had a great night of extra sleep last night, but your body is still dealing with the aftermath of the last *three nights*.

When I have clients or audience members press me on this, I give them the full answer: If you try to sleep ten hours night after night, eventually you will no longer be able to sleep as long because you'll be as caught up as you can get. It won't take you all year to sleep off a year's worth of sleep debt because your body doesn't hold the debt that long. If you sleep ten hours nightly for a week, it will get harder and harder to continue sleeping ten hours.

In fact, it will likely take you less than a week to sleep off your sleep debt unless you are sick or have an underlying health problem or sleep disorder. That means if you are sleeping ten hours night after night for weeks, you should probably consult with your doctor about your health because you may be fighting something off or dealing with a sleep disorder that has no other obvious symptoms.

Remember, this doesn't mean that you have had no consequences for inadequate sleep before catching up. Steve still had the fender bender, didn't get his pan back, and probably caught John's cold. But if he spent the following week getting extra sleep every night, he would finish that second week caught up.

Take me up on it! Get your extra sleep. Track your sleep and how you feel.

### More About Sleep Debt: If I Sleep In on Saturday, Why Do I Feel Exhausted All Day?

I get a version of this question nearly every time I give a talk, and believe me, I've been there myself. Here's the setup: You've had a busy week, a stressful week, or a week where you couldn't get the sleep you needed night after night. For many people, this is a typical week. By the end of it, you're running on fumes. Then comes the weekend—you finally get the chance to crash, you sleep in, maybe ten hours or more. And yet, instead of feeling restored, you wake up groggy and dragging. Why does this happen?

**Simple answer:** You haven't slept enough. Here's how it works.

First, before we start assuming anything, we have to confirm you don't have a sleep disorder like OSA, narcolepsy, or restless limb movement disorder. Also, a blood test will confirm that your thyroid is functioning and you don't have Lyme disease, mononucleosis, or anemia. If we can assume you are not dealing with any of these things, we can start to consider why a healthy person, with healthy sleep, feels exhausted after sleeping.

Let's say your body needs eight hours per night on average. Over the past week you got six hours per night Sunday through Thursday night. That leaves you a sleep debt of ten hours. Then on Friday night you are exhausted from your stressful week with too little sleep. You go to bed a little early and sleep three hours longer. You wake Saturday morning after ten glorious hours of sleep, and you congratulate yourself on a job well done. Shoot, you should be good to go for the weekend, right?

If you do the math, you realize you have only slept off two of your ten hours of sleep debt. Your body hasn't gotten back what it lost. It's like when you are very, very thirsty and you get one glass of water. It feels amazing to drink that glass, but your body wants and needs more than that.

**Longer answer:** You haven't slept enough, AND you are really relaxed. The other side of the question is, Why, after sleeping ten hours, are you feeling even more tired than you had the day before when you were on your fifth day of six hours of sleep?

First, it's Saturday. There is less stress for most people on Saturday, so it's easier to feel more relaxed. Second, by sleeping ten hours last night, you showed your brain that you have the time and ability to sleep much longer than you have been. Remember, your brain is looking for clues like this every day. Sleeping especially long will signal to your brain that it's a rest day. Your brain will respond accordingly. Your brain will also attempt to signal your body to look for more opportunities to rest. The logic goes like this: "Okay, body, we were able to catch up on sleep last night, so today will be more of a rest day. What if we rested some more? Maybe a nap after lunch?" This is how your body and your brain take care of you and take signals from your life to respond and encourage you to take care of yourself.

## Even More About Sleep Debt: Why Is It So Hard to Wake Up on Monday Mornings?

You may remember Ben's story about learning how much sleep he needed. His experience gives me a good place to start to answer this question.

The bottom line for most people is that they have difficulty waking up on Monday mornings because Sunday mornings are treated as an extended "sleep-in" period. When you wake for the day on Sunday morning at 11:00 a.m. and intend to wake up on Monday morning at 7:30 a.m., your body is not ready for the three-and-a-half-hour change.

Remember that our bodies look for clues every day about when things should be happening. Your body uses activities like getting your day started, eating, drinking, using the bathroom, and getting sleepy for bed as clues for when to raise and lower your body temperature, when to get the digestive tract up and running, when to help it close for the night, and so many other things.

When we travel to different time zones for work or vacation, we experience jet lag. What is jet lag? It's the experience that we are hungry at the wrong time, sleepy at the wrong time, and basically misaligned with the new time zone we are in. The more time zones from home you travel, the more you'll feel this. If you travel north or south without crossing time zones, you will feel this *much* less. (It's still a bit discombobulating if you travel long distances, but jet lag won't add to the discomfort if you are traveling in the same time zone.)

What if you only travel one time zone away from home? Do you feel that? You do, but only a little. It's a mild change, and after about twenty-four hours, our bodies adjust to the new time. Our bodies can accommodate about one hour of time zone changes per twenty-four hours,[29] according to research on jet lag. For example, if you travel from Washington, DC, to Kansas City on Friday, that one-hour change in time zones will be something your body is comfortable with by Sunday night.

Your current weekends are a mini version of time zone travel every week. When you sleep in on Sunday until 11:30 a.m. and then try to wake up at 7:30 a.m. on Monday, you are confusing your body almost as much as traveling four time zones west for the weekend and trying to resume normal life on Monday. Sounds challenging, right? It is. Truth is, many of us do this every weekend.

From what you just learned, you now know that an extra four hours of sleep on Sunday morning also means that it will be about four days before your brain will be accustomed to the new (normal) time zone. By Thursday you are all set with the new schedule of sleep and wake. Unfortunately, that gives you one night to use your body's natural circadian rhythm to guide your sleep and wake. When you sleep in on Saturday morning, you've essentially just sent your circadian rhythm on vacation again. Then the process starts all over.

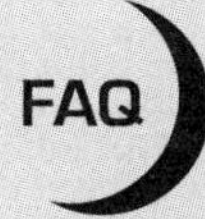


### TO GO DEEP ON SLEEP: How much sleep do you get, Dr. Wolgast?

Touché.

Only recently have audience members started asking me this question, and I appreciate it. It's one thing to listen to someone who knows what they are talking about as they tell you how to live your life, how to eat, how to sleep, or how to train your dog. But if they don't follow their own advice, how much do you trust their words of wisdom?

The short answer is that my sweet spot for sleep is between 7 hours and 15 minutes and 7 hours and 45 minutes per night, and I tend to be a late-morning type of person. That means I'm not really a morning person, and I'm not a night owl. But give me a couple of hours after I wake up, and I'm at my best.

The long answer is that how much sleep I get and how much I need depends on so many things. I am not a robot; I respond to distress, emotion, getting cut off in traffic, catching a cold, overeating, overexercising, and so many other things. Because, like you, I am human.

I have a poor night of sleep every couple of weeks. I know that if I have a super great night of sleep and sleep longer than usual, I will probably sleep shorter than usual the following night or two. On the other hand, I know if I have a poor night of sleep or sleep shorter than usual one night, I will probably sleep longer than usual (or at least more soundly) the following night or two. I trust my body to manage this balance, and my body follows through. I also know that if I consistently provide my body with about 7 hours and 30 minutes of sleep most nights, I will maintain my alertness, my health, and my sense of well-being.

There was a time in my life when I had insomnia. It wasn't long ago. My job was very stressful (I was overseeing a group of about twenty clinicians), and there were multiple demands on my time, my input, my empathy, and my analytic mind. I realized I had insomnia when I was awake at three o'clock in the morning for the third night in a row, making lists of emails and points that I needed to make in meetings. I realized this had become my new normal. I had been waking from sleep or not falling asleep more days than not for months. As a sleep professional, I knew what to do to minimize the daytime impacts and maximize the sleep I was getting, which helped tremendously.

Because I knew the impetus for my insomnia was directly related to my job, and that my job wouldn't be changing in any helpful ways any time soon, I took steps to address the problem. I spoke about my concerns and my limitations with my supervisor, who was incredibly supportive. I talked about finding a different job with my partner and my family. Just opening up and starting that process took much of the pressure off and helped rebalance my sleep.

If you found your job so stressful for months on end that you developed chronic insomnia, would you quit? Why or why not? What goes into that equation for you? You may be wondering if that would be my recommendation to anyone with work stress–induced insomnia. The answer is no. I had great options for other work at the time, and I knew I could step away from this job that didn't suit me for another one that did. That's not the case for everyone or every job. There are always many layers to factors when making major life decisions. If circumstances required me to stay in that job, I would have retooled my evenings using Camping In to work better for me, my relaxation, and my sleep, and I would have gotten through it.

CHAPTER 3

# GOLD MEDAL SLEEP

*You Can Medal on Your Way to Better Sleep*

Before I teach you how to "camp in" to reset your sleep, I am going to provide you with my top twelve tips for sleep health that strengthen your circadian rhythms, boost your chronobiology, and provide the backbone or the scaffolding for the Camping In experience. The tips we're covering include the following:

1. Embrace your mornings.
2. Learn to experience downtime (stop your racing mind!).
3. Make your bedroom your sleep haven.
4. Get in bed with a sleepy brain.
5. Calm your body in bed.
6. Get moving immediately after your alarm goes off.
7. Build the sleep pressure.
8. Now that you've built sleep pressure, keep it!
9. Take control of your phone, your amazing phone.
10. Manage your mind after midnight.

11. Don't believe everything you think.
12. Learn to talk back.

Remember, each of these is part of the Camping-In process (which we'll cover in detail in part four), but each can be used every day of the year, too. Camping In resets your sleep through retraining your body and your brain, using the signals from the world around you and inside of you to guide your drive for sleep. You will spend more time outdoors, have less screen time, and use the sun to help you wake up. The best part of these tips is that not only do they make Camping In effective, but they also can be used every day, generally for free, and each one will support your journey toward better sleep. You won't need to buy much of anything, but there will be decisions to make about how prepared you are to commit to the changes. In the following sections, we'll dive deeper into each tip.

### The Cesar Millan Rule for Sleep Tips

To help you consider how to make sleep-related behavior and lifestyle changes, I want to introduce an idea. I want you to think of my suggestions like a dog owner would think about calling Cesar Millan.

In the early 2000s, Cesar Millan burst into our living rooms as "The Dog Whisperer," with a TV show, several books, and speaking appearances. And he is still out there helping families with their dogs.

Cesar Millan trains the worst, most aggressive dogs to be responsible, family-friendly dogs. His tactics are often intense but only as intense as the situation calls for. Some of the dogs he helps are very aggressive, very anxious, or both.

My point is, not every dog owner needs to call Cesar Millan. If your dog has a bad day or doesn't like getting their toenails trimmed, you don't need to call Cesar Millan. But if your children are afraid of your dog biting them, or you aren't allowed out of the house when your partner is home with the dog because of the dog's aggression, call Cesar.

It's the same with my recommendations here. The worse your sleep is, the more you should consider my recommendations. The better your sleep or the less you worry about your sleep, the more you can consider whether these tips will fit into your life. You be the judge.

## LET'S GET STARTED WITH GOLD MEDAL SLEEP!

If changing your relationship with sleep were easy, I wouldn't have a job. I want you to consider making changes to your sleep life on a scale that fits you and your life. If you want to make a small change in your sleep behaviors, go for bronze. You have medaled! If you are looking for a stretch goal, aim for silver—you have done more than most and are up to the challenge! And if you are looking to reshape your sleep at the highest level, go for gold! Every medal wins in my book. Every change takes commitment and effort. And arriving at the bronze level may be plenty for you, or it could inspire you to push for the next level.

Choose your goals based on what area of your sleep or daytime routine offers the greatest opportunity for improvement, the area that seems to speak to you most directly or that you have been told is your weak spot. And choose goals that are doable for you; I want you to experience success. That means if you've struggled with sleep problems for years, starting with goals in the bronze realm is a smart start. You can always take things a step higher after you've had some initial success and enjoyed the improvements that come along with it. There is a billion-dollar *Sleep Better Now!* industry and your old habits working against you. Be good to yourself—you deserve good sleep, and you can get there—just don't be in too big of a rush. And remember that every night is another chance to medal. You don't have to figure it all out tonight—you get the rest of your life to work on medaling.

## THE RHYTHMS OF BEING HUMAN

In fourth-grade natural science class with Ms. Nothern, I learned that raccoons and wolves are nocturnal, and I am not. My mind was blown! I could not believe that some animals think of nighttime the same way we think of daytime: the time to be up and around, taking care of chores, seeing friends, and playing with toys. What we didn't get into is that the determination of being diurnal (daytime alert animals) or nocturnal (like the raccoons) is built into our DNA. It means that our brains are hardwired with many systems designed to keep us asleep at night and alert in the day. These systems are collectively called our chronobiology, or circadian rhythms.

In a nutshell, circadian rhythms are a host of internal clocks in our bodies that operate to keep us on a schedule. When they work, they help our bodies know when to sleep, when to feel sharp and active, when to feel hungry (and not hungry), when to use the bathroom, and when to be relaxed.

Do circadian rhythms prevent humans from staying up all night? No. Does this mean raccoons and deer are unable to walk around in the daytime? Again, no. But it does mean that our bodies are more effective when we follow the circadian rhythms in our DNA. We live longer when we stay in our chronobiological lane: sleeping when it's dark and being active when it's light.

These internal clocks rely on the world outside of us and our own actions to run smoothly. While the drive to be diurnal is hardwired, your circadian rhythms look for cues every day to keep the beat. Your activities have a lot to do with how smoothly they run. My suggestions here are going to all be because you are human, you are diurnal, and there are many innate human systems that we can reinforce to promote healthy sleep patterns.

## Tip#1 Embrace the Morning

Mornings set the tone for everything that follows in your day. The way you wake up, the light you see, and the consistency of your habits act as powerful signals to your brain and body about how to function. Think of it as giving your internal orchestra its cue: When you rise at the same time, your circadian rhythms begin playing in sync, preparing you for alertness, energy, focus, and, eventually, restful sleep. This section is about learning how to embrace your mornings with intention so that your nights can become more restorative and your days more productive. Let's look at some specific techniques to achieve that.

### Wake Up at the Same Time Every Day and Get Your Day Started

If there is one thing you use from this book and nothing else, make it this one.

When you wake up and start your day, you restart several internal body clocks. It's like turning on the engine for the car. You may have packed the trunk for your trip last night, but the car won't start the day's journey until the engine is running. Starting your day initiates dozens of circadian rhythms, from your brain to your gut. And doing it at a consistent time makes for a smooth-running engine.

There is one internal clock that operates like a sand timer—the kind where you flip it over, and the sand drains from the top half to the bottom. When you start your day, you flip the sand timer, and about fifteen hours later the sand will run out. When the sand runs out, your brain will send neurochemicals to signal that it is time to start settling down for sleep.

**Q: Why wake up at the same time every day?**

A: Your brain is a pattern-recognition machine; it is hungry for patterns and looks for them all the time. There are many circadian rhythms that are seeking daily patterns for wake time, bedtime, mealtime, and so on. If you wake at 10:00 a.m. on Saturday and Sunday and then 6:45 a.m. on Monday, you have confused this part of your brain—it thought you were going to sleep three more hours! The clinical name for this is *social jet lag*, but I like to call it *weekend jet lag*. For college students with variable daily schedules, it's often more like waking up in a different time zone every day.

**Q: Will this work if I just wake up at the same time but lie quietly in bed for a while?**
A: Not as well. When your alarm goes off, just get moving. If you lie still after waking, the part of your brain looking for patterns isn't going to know if you are up for the day or if you are preparing to return to sleep. Get up, get moving, and make the message clear.

Now it's time for the medal recommendations. After each of these tips, I will provide a gold-, silver-, and bronze-level technique for you to choose from. These will provide you with a ladder of options, from least effort to most. Don't get hung up on the three I provide you—there are more than three ways to do all my tips. Make the way you choose fit you and your lifestyle. Make it challenge you in a way that you believe you can accomplish.

## RECOMMENDATIONS

Based on these ideas, here are my recommendations for maintaining a consistent wake time:

- **Bronze:** Pick your Monday–Friday wake time and stick to it. When the alarm goes off, get moving within fifteen minutes. On Saturday, sleep in an extra two hours and enjoy it. On Sunday, sleep in an extra hour and enjoy it. On Monday morning, experience just a one-hour jet lag experience.
- **Silver:** Pick your Monday–Friday wake time and stick to it. When the alarm goes off, get moving within fifteen minutes. On Saturday, sleep in an extra hour and enjoy it. On Sunday, sleep in an extra thirty minutes and enjoy it. On Monday morning, experience something short of a time zone change.
- **Gold:** Pick your Monday–Friday wake time and stick to it *seven* days per week. When the alarm goes off, get moving within fifteen minutes. Enjoy Monday morning feeling like every other day rather than "Monday morning." After two weeks of consistent morning waking, pay attention to how much easier it is to get started with your day.

## STOP USING YOUR SNOOZE ALARM (ENJOY DISNEY WORLD!)

The snooze alarm is an invention created by people who did not understand how sleep works. If you had the choice between sleeping an extra twenty minutes or being awakened three times during the same twenty minutes, which would you choose? If you prefer being awakened by your alarm, you are kidding yourself.

If you are following the first recommendation, this one comes easily. Waking up at the same time every day means just that. Fiddling with your snooze alarm only delays waking and weakens your internal clocks. In addition, the more consistently you hit snooze when you hear the alarm go off, the more your brain associates the sound of the alarm with snoozing rather than waking up. Remember, your circadian rhythms are looking for cues every day to keep the beat. One of the strongest cues is the time you wake up and start your day.

Most people I have met use a snooze alarm. I did it for years, too. It feels so good to hit snooze and go back to sleep. It just isn't good sleep.

Let me compare your night of sleep to a trip to Disney World. Remember that sleep happens in four stages that follow a consistent pattern:

- Stage 1 is light sleep.
- Stage 2 continues light sleep while transitioning from light to deep sleep.
- Stage 3 is deep sleep and is what most people experience as the heaviest sleep.
- REM is the final stage of sleep, where most dreaming happens.

Sleep cycles follow a consistent pattern across the night, with differences in how long each stage lasts that depend on how long one has been asleep. Each cycle of sleep follows this pattern:

**Stage 1 → Stage 2 → Stage 3 → Stage 2 → REM**

We spend most of our time at night in the transitional stage 2 sleep before and after stage 3 and before REM sleep. While all stages are important, the stages of sleep that provide the clearest benefits are stage 3 and REM sleep. Deep sleep and REM are the stages that your body will demand from you the longer you have been awake. Sleep professionals use brain activity to determine what stage of sleep you are in.

Back to Disney World. The parts of Disney World that are awesome are the rides, and they are inside the gates. But you don't just get out of your car and walk through the gates; you take the tram, bus, or boat from the parking lot to the gates. Imagine the tram of your sleep is light sleep (stages 1 and 2). You need the tram to get to the rides, but the tram isn't the reason you came to Disney World, and light sleep isn't the reason you want more sleep.

When your alarm goes off, you are instantly pulled from the rides in Disney (most likely REM sleep) back to your car. When you hit the snooze alarm, you hop back on the tram to get inside. About the time you are getting inside the park and to the rides (the more meaningful sleep you crave), your alarm goes off again.

Hit snooze. Get back on the tram. Repeat.

Let's imagine you can sit down with your ten-year-old self:

Present you: Let's say you are in Disney World.

Ten-year-old you: I like where this is going.

Present you: You are on the rides, and you've been there all day.

Ten-year-old you: Are you sending me to Disney? You're awesome!

Present you: It's almost time to leave, but you have twenty more minutes.

Ten-year-old you: How many more rides can I go on before we have to leave?

Present you: Wait, here's my question: Would you rather ride the tram back and forth from the parking lot or stay in the park and keep riding the rides?

Ten-year-old you: What? Why are you asking me that?

Present you: Just answer the question.
Ten-year-old you: Um, yeah. I would stay on the rides. Are you okay? Do you need to see a doctor? That's the dumbest question I've ever heard. Am I going to think this is a good question when I'm your age?

## RECOMMENDATIONS

Here are my recommendations for cutting back on snoozing and starting your mornings with more clarity:

- **Bronze:** Allow yourself a low number of "snooze away" passes for each week. I suggest aiming for two or three per week, but the number you choose is up to you. Then use those passes judiciously based on how desperate you feel for a little more shut-eye.
- **Silver:** Allow yourself to rest quietly with your eyes open in bed for five minutes before getting started. This isn't snoozing; it is starting your morning more gently. You are awake in bed without looking at your phone for a few minutes.
- **Gold:** Get out of bed and start your day right away every day. Also, consider sleeping with the blinds open so that the sun will help wake you for the day. When your friends wonder why you are so consistent every day, you can share this tip with them.

## GO INTO THE LIGHT (NO, NOT THAT LIGHT)

Your alarm has gone off, you didn't jump back on the tram, and you are out of bed. Congratulations! Now it's time to get near a window or go outside. This is a big piece of Camping In.

Your brain has internal clocks waiting to see the first glimpse of sunlight. This clock works in tandem with the hourglass timer I mentioned earlier. The first significant light of the day starts a countdown timer to bedtime. When that timer ends, you will get a neurochemical boost that encourages sleepiness.

Even more—the first sunlight of the day will help awaken you, and the more time you spend near a window or outdoors, the stronger your circadian rhythms will operate. It's buy one, get one free! It's not the brightness that does it—it doesn't matter if the sun is shining or it's raining cats and dogs; it's the blue light waves that come from the sun.

First, the blue light signals your brain that it's time to get up and start your day. Then, sunlight throughout your day strengthens that signal and encourages alertness. This alertness eventually wears off in the late afternoon, and a dip in energy is a new signal to another circadian rhythm that evening is coming soon. Think of sunlight first thing in the morning as a boost to starting your day and sunlight the rest of the day as a boost to getting your body ready for bed.

### Let's Go Outside!

Your brain and body are built to read the sunlight and darkness for cues on how to operate. The system still works even if you are living in a cave with no access to anything related to sunlight but not as well. How do we know that? Because researchers Nathanial Kleitman and his graduate student Bruce Richardson in 1938, and later Michel Siffre spent weeks and months in a cave without any sunlight or access to any day or night cues, and when they finished, they were still essentially operating on a twenty-four-hour day[30] (a few minutes more than that, but what's a few minutes difference when you are living in a cave?). Other researchers have done this and obtained the same result.[31] That's pretty good for a circadian system that has no sun guidance. What works better than living in a cave with no sunlight? Allowing the sun and the darkness to let your brain know when it is time to sleep and wake.

If you search the internet, you will read that all you need for your daily dose of sunlight is about fifteen minutes. More specifically, you should be outdoors or near a window where the sun is bright during morning daylight hours for about fifteen minutes. More than fifteen minutes is better, but fifteen minutes is enough to signal your circadian rhythms. Sunlight is what our bodies are designed to read and understand, but artificial blue light is better than nothing. I'll talk more about using an artificial blue light in the next section for those who need it.

The vital piece of this is the blue wavelength of light, or blue light. You've heard about this as the enemy emanating from your screens—phones, laptops, TVs, etc. And that's true (sort of—more later). But blue light is sleep's best friend during the day.

Deep in your brain is an area called the suprachiasmatic nuclei (SCN), which is the ruler of your many circadian rhythms. Every day and every night the SCN looks for confirmatory information about your daily rhythms.

Let me pull this all together. For starting your day and preparing to do your daytime activities, the SCN pays attention to what time you eat (especially your first food), what time in the day you first use the bathroom (especially number two), what time your heart rate reflects that you are moving around and not just trying to get back to sleep, and so on. The most important morning cue to your SCN is what time of day you get your first daylight in your eyes[32] (again, at least fifteen minutes, though more is better).

For ending your day and preparing for sleep, the SCN pays attention to what time you stop eating, the last time your heart rate reflects doing more than just relaxing, and so on. But the most critical cue to your SCN for sleep is what time you experienced your last strong blue light as well as how much time you spent outside during the day. Later in the book, I'll share more about evening blue light exposure.

In summary: get sunlight. The more sunlight you get, the better your body regulates your day and your night. You don't even have to go outside to get it—windows work well, so if you can't be outdoors, find a window. Sunlight remains free and is available every day because the clouds cannot prevent blue light from coming through.

The time we spend outdoors has shrunk over the last seventy-five years. When my parents were children, few indoor activities could hold a kid's attention the way running around the neighborhood with friends and a ball could. For thousands of years, even as recently as your grandparents' era, much of the work was done outdoors. Construction and farming were common occupations with large percentages of Americans undertaking them. A research group called Building H (the *H* is for *health*) surveyed thousands of Americans in 2020 and found that about 37% of adults spend less than thirty minutes outdoors most days. Women spend less time outdoors than men, and younger adults spend less time outdoors than older adults. Nearly 60% of American adults spend less than an hour outdoors daily.[33]

It wasn't long ago that this would have been unthinkable. In 1900, the majority of American workers were employed in outdoor, agricultural, and construction-based jobs, and as a result American adults averaged as much as six hours per day outdoors.[34] Much of that was working, but even those Americans who worked indoors would spend leisure time outdoors. What accounts for the biggest change?

We work indoors, and weather (both hot and cold) drives us indoors. Seventy-five years ago, hot weather meant it was warmer indoors than outdoors ("At least there is a breeze outside!"). Today, most homes and nearly all businesses have air conditioning, and as a result, our bodies aren't adept at spending hours outside.

What changed is that being indoors became more comfortable and more entertaining. Our screens are easiest to use indoors—no glare, smaller chance of rain on the electronics, etc. Our jobs have us working indoors most of the daytime, and some of us are working two jobs, even three, all indoors. There are far fewer farmers than there used to be due to technology and corporate farming. We still have construction workers, but again, the machines we use for construction mean fewer construction workers are outdoors because machines do the work of many workers.

The outdoors is just that—out the door. It doesn't cost anything to walk outside the door of your home. For the purposes of your sleep, your health, and your mental health, just getting outside for the low price of free is all that is needed. There is no need to buy exercise equipment, specialized outdoor clothing, or even sunglasses (you'll get more blue light without the sunglasses). For the sake of your circadian rhythms, just step outside in an area that is sunny for fifteen minutes first thing in the morning. Then step outside again later to boost those rhythms and help your body prepare for sleep.

## RECOMMENDATIONS

Here are my recommendations for getting more sunlight:

- **Bronze:** Upon waking up for the day, open your blinds and spend fifteen minutes sitting near a sun-facing window while eating breakfast or getting ready for your day.
- **Silver:** Do the bronze activity and then, at least three days a week, spend an additional hour outside during

the day. Maybe one day you'll take a walk; another day you'll sit outside to eat lunch. You could even phone a friend or check your email while sitting outside. (Daytime screentime is okay, and doing it outdoors is a double win for your circadian rhythms.)

- **Gold:** Do the bronze activity each morning. Then, during the day, at least five days a week, spend two hours outside. You could use that time to walk to and from work or the grocery store, exercise, or visit a neighbor if you want to be productive with your time. But you could also meet a friend for a chat or a coffee outdoors, take a hike, or enjoy watching the sunset. Consider finding a friend to join you in this effort.

## WAIT! WHAT ABOUT THOSE OF US IN CANADA, MAINE, OR ALASKA?

Sunlight is sunlight unless you live far from the equator. In that case, sunlight is more seasonal. There is a reason that the growing seasons in Alaska and the Scandinavian countries are very short: The sun only shines for most of the day for half the year. Those of you who live near the equator may have never experienced the inconsistency of the day/night schedule that millions of people in the far northern and far southern hemispheres have. In fact, people closer to the north and south poles have been developing techniques to deal with the short days of winter for as long as they have lived there.

Does this mean people who live in Iceland or Alaska have weaker circadian rhythms? Absolutely not. Remember the researchers I mentioned who lived in a cave for a month to see how their bodies would react? They kept their circadian rhythms without any sunlight. The rhythms weren't strong, but they were consistent. And even near the poles there is some light most days, even in winter.

My son and I visited Iceland in early February a few years ago to see the northern lights. The people there were kind and easygoing. They were warm and friendly. They weren't sleep deprived and acted like their circadian rhythms were intact. The sun came up just after ten o'clock each morning, and it was setting just after five o'clock each evening. How do they manage? Human bodies and brains are flexible, and the culture and mindset around engaging and enjoying winter make it easier for Icelanders to not only maintain solid circadian rhythms but also enjoy the winter months. Kari Leibowitz's *How to Winter* is a fantastic book that outlines her research and explains how the cultures of the dark winters not only survive but thrive. Danish and Norwegians use the word *hygge* to describe feeling cozy and happy, and it translates well into the dark winter months. I encourage the people I work with to adopt a mindset that embraces colder, darker weather as time for relaxing, reading, candlelight, and getting cozy while making the most of the sunlight when they can.

Sunlight is king of the circadian rhythms but don't forget the other royalty. If you are living far north or far south (Argentina and Scandinavia, I'm talking to you here), your process of staying on a healthy daily rhythm will rely more on activity and meal timing, the queen and prince of the circadian rhythms. The more consistent you can be with your wake times and your mealtimes, especially your earliest meals, the easier it will be for your circadian rhythms to inform your body about sleep timing.

Think about this as having a person in your head who operates your internal clocks. There's a wrinkle: This person generally knows what to do but has a memory of only about three or four days. This person wakes up with you every day and begins to look for clues about what time of day it is. Every day! And you supply the clues through your sunlight exposure, your mealtimes, and your activity. When you live very far north or south, winter means this clock operator is more desperate for those other clues because the sunlight is briefer. In this scenario, it is important to double down on what you can control.

If you live in Alaska or Edmonton, you won't have a lot of sunlight during January. But the times of the day when there is sunlight should be taken advantage of. Get out there or at least sit near a window because it's cold outside. Does driving or sitting in a car count for circadian clue-giving? Yes, because cars have 360 degrees of windows (extra credit for a moonroof), and if you are driving, fewer things block the sun rays from your vision.

*What if I live in Nova Scotia, and I need to be at work before the sun comes up and go home after the sun goes down? How am I going to get my daylight?* One of the advantages of living in the modern world is that we can access inexpensive electric blue light. It's not as effective as the sun, but it's much more effective than having no sunlight.

Light boxes, blue lights, or SAD (seasonal affective disorder) lamps have been around for a couple of decades. Blue light lamps used to cost well over $1,000 and were large, sometimes as big as a table. Today, you can choose from a variety of smaller blue light lamps for prices below $25 and in sizes small enough to carry in your purse or backpack. They also come in the form of some very space-age-looking glasses (e.g., AYO, Luminette—but do not wear these while driving). There are many reliable manufacturers out there for these lamps and glasses. Look for *10,000 lux* as the marker for standard strength and choose something that will fit your lifestyle.

Once you have your lamp, the goal is to use it for at least fifteen minutes as soon as your intended wake time arrives for the day. You don't have to look at it; it just needs to be in your field of vision for these fifteen minutes. It's okay to look away, blink, or walk away to get your socks and come back.

Where do you use it? I recommend to many of my insomnia patients, and those who live in northern zones, that they find the easiest place to use their blue light lamp every day and park it there. Breakfast table? Bathroom sink? Your desk at work? All of these are good. And the best spot is the one you will be able to use with the most consistency. Get in a routine for using it and stick with it.

Who shouldn't use it? If you take medication that makes you sensitive to bright light—such as some antibiotics, certain antipsychotics, or St. John's Wort—this may not be for you. If you have any chronic health issues related to your eyes, it's best to discuss using blue light treatment with your doctor. In addition, if you have been diagnosed with bipolar disorder, or have a family history of bipolar disorder, talk with your doctor and your mental health care provider before using blue light. Because blue light works to enhance your circadian rhythms, overuse or misuse of blue light can encourage manic episodes, which no one wants. People with photosensitive epilepsy seem to tolerate blue light without problems, because it's not the sort of light that can cause seizures. But I encourage those people to speak with their neurologist before starting blue-light use.

## RECOMMENDATIONS

Here are my recommendations for getting enough light during winters far from the equator:

- **Bronze:** Upon waking up for the day, open your blinds and spend fifteen minutes with a 10,000 lux blue-light lamp while eating breakfast or getting ready for your day.
- **Silver:** Do the bronze activity, and then, at least three days a week, spend an added hour outside during the hours after sunrise. Maybe one day you'll take a walk; another

day you'll sit outside to eat lunch. You could even phone a friend or check your email while sitting outside (daytime screentime is okay!). If it's too cold for these activities, do them while sitting near a sun-facing window. In the evenings, relax and enjoy the calmer evening energy with some candlelight and a craft project or a card game.

- **Gold:** Do the bronze activity each morning. Then, during the day at least five days a week, spend two hours outside or sitting near a sun-facing window. You could use that time to walk to and from work or the grocery store, exercise, or visit a neighbor if you want to be productive with your time. But you could also meet a friend for a chat or a coffee, take a hike, or enjoy watching the sunset. Consider finding a friend to join you in this effort to make follow-through more likely. In the evenings, lean into your local cozy culture—enjoy some candlelight and storytelling or read a book with your favorite blanket.

Now that you have started your day without a snooze alarm at the same time as yesterday and you've gotten into the sunlight, your chronobiological success story is underway! Let's work on more techniques to make your daytime activities help your nighttime sleep.

## TIP #2: LEARN TO EXPERIENCE DOWNTIME AND STOP THE RACING MIND!

In the past several years, the number of people seeking my professional help with the complaint "I can't turn my mind off at night" has increased significantly. This was something I heard occasionally prior to 2010, but now it's so common that I always expect to hear it from my clients.

Khalid and I met because he was struggling to fall asleep, needing nearly two hours to settle in for his night. "I can't turn my brain off. I turn out the lights, and it's like something in my brain turns on. The only way I can stop it is to watch YouTube videos of Russian dash cams," he told me. The point he was missing is that by spending free moments engaging with his phone throughout the day—not just the last minutes before trying to sleep—he was keeping his brain busy, and it couldn't simply turn off when he wanted to sleep.

Here is a short list of some of the most common reasons your thoughts might be racing at bedtime:

- Instagram
- TikTok
- Reddit
- Twitter/X
- texts
- games you've downloaded (*Candy Crush*, solitaire, etc.)
- emails
- online shopping
- gambling apps
- pornography
- whatever has become popular since this book was written

Your brain needs time to rest. Giving your brain downtime doesn't mean peacefully meditating on an empty beach. It could be while you are walking from one place to another, while sitting for a few minutes after you eat a meal or watch a show, or while pausing during almost any activity, anywhere, anytime. It simply requires letting your mind run on its own without shoving content into it from your devices.

Based on my work with my clients, especially those who are heavy digital media users, if you don't allow your brain time to run freely, it will find its own time and force you to think about the things it believes are important. The one time every day that everyone experiences free time is the time just before falling asleep. The less time you allow your brain to do its own thing all day, with no digital content coming in, the more likely you are to spend the time between deciding to go to sleep and sleeping with your mind running.

Here is how I encourage my clients to think about their devices: I tell them the more engaging the device, or activity on the device, the more downtime they should prepare for. The keyword here is *engaging*. Watching a television show, even a good one, engages your brain less than playing a video game on your phone, even a bad one. That is because, in a video game, you are controlling the action, not passively watching the screen. And video games that are on a system (Xbox, PlayStation, Switch) are more engaging than games on your phone, even a good phone. **Lesson one: Playing games is more engaging than scrolling social media, and social media is more engaging than watching shows.**

On your devices, passive content that refreshes often is more *engaging* than content that holds a storyline. For example, to your brain, TikTok is more engaging than your emails. Shopping may be more engaging than Instagram. Instagram is more engaging than Reddit. *Candy Crush* is more engaging than all of them, and *Zelda* or *Mario Kart* is more engaging than *Candy Crush*.

If you are looking to diminish your brain-racing at bedtime, reduce your brain busyness while you are awake by disengaging. I'm not trying to break up you and your phone, but I do think you two should spend a little more time apart, especially in the evenings. Give your brain a break. Consider reading a book, talking—not texting—with a friend, playing a board game, or doing a crossword or word search.

I know, I know. I sound like your grandfather right now. But guess what? Back in Gramp's day, there was a lot less insomnia and a whole lot fewer racing brains.

There will be more discussion and recommendations about phone use in my eighth tip.

## RECOMMENDATIONS

Here are my recommendations for reducing a busy brain at night:

- **Bronze:** Give yourself five to ten minutes during the day to think about whatever comes to mind while all screens are away and on silent. Do this somewhere that is not your bed or bedroom.
- **Silver:** Give yourself five to ten minutes at two separate times during the day to think about whatever comes to mind while all screens are away and on silent. Do this while outside or sitting near a window, maybe while taking a walk.
- **Gold:** Give yourself five to ten minutes at least three separate times during the day to think about whatever comes to mind while all screens are away and on silent. At least one of those times, do this while outside or sitting near a window, maybe while taking a walk.

## TIP #3: MAKE YOUR BEDROOM YOUR SLEEP HAVEN

For many of you, this will seem obvious. But if you've never considered your sleep environment as something that promotes or detracts from sleep, it's time we had a talk.

Your brain is constantly looking for cues about what to do based on where you are. If you look inside the refrigerator long enough, you may start to feel hungry. If you sit in your dentist's waiting room, you become anxious. What I want for you is that when you get into your bed, you begin to relax and maybe even become sleepier. Let's get you set up for the right cues for your brain so that you can have strong signaling.

Let's start with a mantra. The field of insomnia treatment, and specifically *stimulus control techniques for insomnia*, created a mantra to help you: "Sleep is for the bed; the bed is for sleep." That means when you are in bed, you are ready for sleep. It also means you aren't sleeping elsewhere—the couch, your office, or really anywhere else. You are training your brain to sleep in your bed. Two other activities allowed in your bed are sickness and sex. But that's the whole list.

Next, you want your bedroom to be sleep encouraging. There are many things that people keep in their bedrooms that discourage sleep, from phones to clocks, to TVs and so on. I'm going to tackle phones later, so remember that I warned you, but I'll elaborate on the rest here:

- **Clocks:** Can you think of a time you looked at a clock in the middle of the night and thought, "Oh, great. Now I get to sleep more!" If you have, you probably sleep so well that you would never have picked up this book unless you are a friend or family member of mine. If I'm right—thanks for reading this far, even though you are probably tired of me talking to you about sleep! You really are a friend.

But the rest of you are remembering all the times you looked at your bedroom clock and thought, "Ugh. It's already ___ o'clock. And now I only have ___ hours left to get some sleep." Does that sound like a good way to promote sleep? It's not.

- **TVs:** You've already heard how the twenty-four-hour news cycle changed how people slept in the 1980s. Now there are infinite channels and content to watch, not to mention the video game systems you can use through your TV (which I'll dive into more later). TVs are not sleep encouraging; they are engaging, and they belong in other places in your home.
- **Lighting:** The lighting in your bedroom should be mild, not blinding. A good rule of thumb is to use lights that aren't halogen, are covered by lampshades, and are soft.
- For lighting when you wake in the night, consider getting motion-activated soft lighting under your bed or under a piece of furniture in your bedroom. I stayed in a hotel in Florida once where I stepped out of bed and soft lighting came on, activated by the motion of my feet, and it lit the path to the bathroom. Genius! Why don't we all have something like this? Immediately I bought a set of these lights for my elderly parents. After they had them installed, several of their friends bought them as well. Having motion-activated lights under your bed or dresser means you don't have to turn on the lights

in the night to get to the bathroom, and you don't have to wake your bedpartner either.

- **Bed:** Your bed should be comfortable. It should be something you feel good lying down on. Humans are very different and have different bed needs, so I'm not going to tell you which bed to own—you need to find what works for you. However, if your mattress is more than ten years old, it's probably time for you to find a new bed. Mattresses have a "useful life endpoint," where they eventually wear out and offer you less of the comfort you have enjoyed. And don't ask Google about the microorganisms that will colonize in your mattress after several years; you don't want to know.
- **Noise:** Is it noisy in your bedroom? Does the noise bother you? Can you remove the noise? A squirrel burrowing in your walls can be incredibly frustrating, but there are people who can help you cover the entry points for your squirrel guests. Does your neighbor watch TV loudly late at night? Consider a white-noise machine near the wall that has a timer to shut off after a couple of hours. The more you can do to create a bedroom space that seems inviting and encouraging to sleep, the better.

## RECOMMENDATIONS

Here are my recommendations for creating a sleep haven:

- **Bronze:** Unplug your bedroom TV for one week and put the remote control in your sock drawer along with your clock. Decide if and how you need to manage any distracting or frustrating noises you hear while in your bed.

- **Silver:** Remove your TV and alarm clock from your bedroom entirely. Additionally, ensure you have soft lighting and one lamp, with just one bulb, to light the bedroom while you are preparing for bed. Consider a light bulb built to light a room without blue light (find these on the internet and at big retailers).
- **Gold:** With your TV and clock removed and your soft blue light–free lighting in the evening, you can now add the under-the-bed motion-sensitive lighting and consider whether it's time for a new mattress.

## TIP #4: GET IN BED WITH A SLEEPY BRAIN

Now you are ready for bed. Wait, how did you know? So many people today get into bed when they think it is *time* for bed. Other people monitor their bodies so closely for a sign that they are sleepy that they effectively ward off sleepiness by signaling to their brains that they need to stay alert. And some of the lucky ones just get in bed and fall asleep immediately. It's time to find a middle ground. The goal is to get in bed when your brain is ready to sleep.

If you've ever helped an infant learn to sleep, you know that putting them down when they are wide awake isn't going to do much good. On the other hand, putting them down when they are sound asleep only teaches them to fall asleep while you are holding them. This is a workable solution while they are cute and tiny, but it gets challenging rocking them to sleep when they weigh ninety-five pounds. When parenting an infant, sleep training means looking for the sweet spot—when your baby is sleepy but not asleep. When you do this consistently your baby learns to fall asleep when they get in the crib or bed.

That last paragraph is also about you. You are the baby, but you are also the parent trying to figure out how to get the baby to learn to fall asleep in bed—not wide awake for ninety minutes in bed and not on the couch watching TV.

Healthy, rested adults need ten to fifteen minutes to fall asleep. That's the time it takes for your body to recognize you are in bed, wind down, and drift off. Does it take you much less time? You may not need this section. People who fall asleep very quickly often have a great deal of built-up sleep debt. People who get in bed and need more than half an hour to fall asleep, maybe an hour or two, are my audience here. Let's get better at getting to bed with a sleepy brain.

First, I want you to notice that I'm talking about a sleepy brain. This is different from a tired brain or an exhausted brain. We can be tired all day but not sleepy. We can be physically exhausted without being sleepy. Being sleepy means being ready to fall asleep. I want you to get to bed with a sleepy, ready-to-sleep brain.

What is sleepy? Because we are so busy engaging our brains with exciting content (TikTok, PlayStation, YouTube), we often don't notice the subtle hints our bodies send us to let us know it's time to get to sleep. As a sleep clinician, I often hear clients tell me they don't know when to go to bed because they have no idea what they feel like when they are sleepy.

Let's try something right now for about sixty seconds. I want you to finish reading this paragraph, set this book down, close your eyes, and pay attention to your body. With your eyes shut, does your body feel heavy? Did your eyes close a little too easily? How hard will it be for you to open your eyes again (on a scale of 1 to 10, with 10 being very difficult and 1 being very easy)? Don't open your eyes yet. Next,

I want you to count backward from fifty by threes. Go all the way to zero. And then it is time to open your eyes.

It's time to give this a try. Set the book down and close your eyes. I'll wait for you in the next paragraph.

Seriously. Set the book down. This is why you are here.

Okay, welcome back.

What did you notice? How heavy were your eyes? How heavy did your body feel? What was your estimate for how difficult it would be to open your eyes? And how accurate were you? And how challenging was the counting backward exercise? These are some of the simple features of assessing your level of sleepiness. Being sleepy means difficulty tracking with your eyes and having a slower processing speed for thinking, like when counting backward. Each person experiences fatigue a bit differently, but we all have a slower processing speed when we are sleepy.

My challenge for you, should you choose to accept it, is to assess your sleepiness at least three times daily—early in the day, middle of the day, and around your bedtime. Each time, notice if you are feeling sleepy, not just tired. If you are feeling sleepy and it is bedtime, get to bed. If not, stay out of bed until that time. The longer you stay out of bed, the sleepier you will get; though it could take a while if you struggle with starting to sleep.

## RECOMMENDATIONS

Here are my recommendations for getting to bed with a sleepy brain:

- **Bronze:** Once or twice a week, after your evening meal, sit quietly with your eyes closed for just a minute or two, assessing your sleepiness. Track your progress and how accurate your estimate for opening your eyes was.
- **Silver:** Follow the bronze steps every day.

- **Gold:** Follow the bronze steps a few times daily. The timing is up to you but do it at different times. Notice the changing sleepiness levels across the course of the day and lean into the moments when you are feeling sleepiest. These will guide you to being better at going to bed when you are sleepy—not just at bedtime.

## TIP #5: CALM YOUR BODY IN BED

Congratulations on getting into bed sleepy! You have done half of the hard work. I'm going to assume that the struggle isn't over yet. If you are reading this, you are likely to be someone whose brain isn't clear about how to fall asleep and who can spend several minutes or hours getting from awake to asleep. You are already working on reducing your distracted hours during the day so that your brain knows how to use downtime, but you aren't there yet. That's okay! It takes time and practice. These tips for calming yourself will make Camping In especially useful when we get there.

Even if you are someone who gets into bed sleepy and falls asleep in ten to fifteen minutes, I can provide tips to improve the process. These are tips that I have learned over the years, and there are always others—I can't present everything here. If you have things that work for you, keep doing them! And message me to let me know what they are so I can share them with others.

My goal is for you to improve the transition between being awake and being asleep. It's a normal, natural process. But if you learn to get in the way of falling asleep, you are part of the problem. What I will teach you here is how to get out of the way. And I'll agree with you that it's ironic to teach you to get out of the way of a natural, normal human function. But hey, you have to start somewhere.

This transition is part mental, part biological. Let's focus on your body first.

### Prepare Your Body

Your breath and breathing are very strong signals to your brain and body about your current state. When you are distressed, you breathe more shallowly. When you are more relaxed, you breathe more deeply. That's natural. To encourage your body to be calmer, you can use deep breathing without hyperventilating as a strong signal to your brain that things are good, and the body can relax. That's why when I meet someone who has panic attacks, the first thing we discuss is how to breathe deeply. Breath work isn't new. It's been practiced for thousands of years and studied beyond what our needs are here. Let's start with a simple technique called box breathing. Then use it when you are getting into bed tonight.

### Box Breathing

**Box breathing** is easy to learn because the concept is simple. Even if you've never tried deep breathing, you can start using it tonight. To use box breathing, I want you to close your eyes and imagine you are drawing a box with your breathing. Sit quietly and comfortably and use your finger to draw the lines of the box as you go from step to step on your leg.

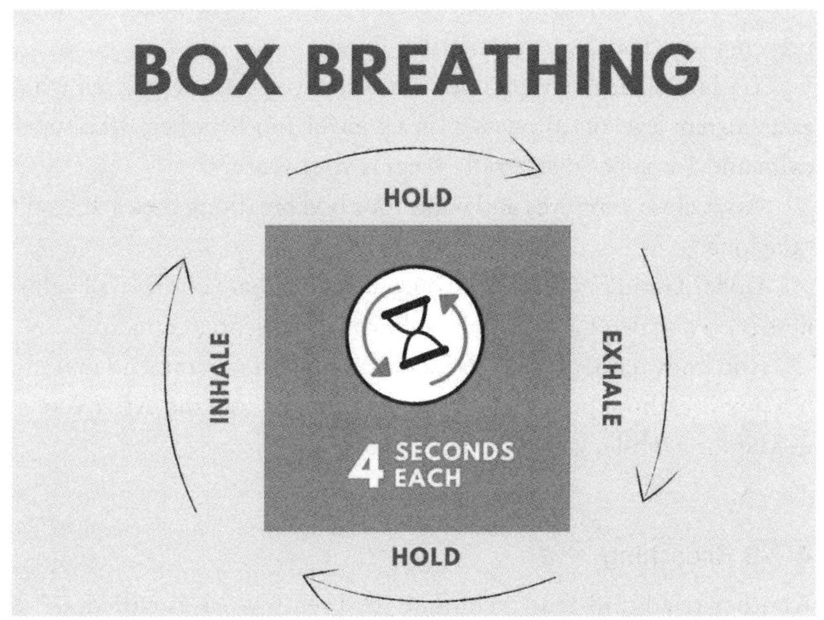


1. **Inhale for four:** Draw a line up while inhaling and counting to four.
2. **Hold for four:** Now draw a line across the top of the box while holding that breath and counting to four.
3. **Exhale for four:** Now draw a line down while slowly exhaling to a count of four.
4. **Rest for four:** Finally, draw a line across the bottom of the box while you rest (don't inhale yet) while counting to four.

See the box? It's fours on all sides. Easy, right?

Holding for four and resting between breaths for four are both very important. Box breathing does two things: First, it helps signal to your brain that you are not in a hurry and you can rest. Second, it prevents you from hyperventilating. Really.

Try box breathing right now. But before you do, ask yourself what your current level of calmness is on a scale of 1 to 10, where 10 is super calm and 1 is super distressed. What is your score?

Now, close your eyes and make four box breathing boxes. It won't take long.

Done? Good practice. Ask yourself again what your level of calmness is on a scale of 1 to 10. How do your two scores compare?

You know enough now to use this tonight. I recommend making ten box-breathing boxes when you get into bed tonight. After you've used it for a while, you can change it up.

### 4-7-8 Breathing

Another tried-and-true technique for breath work is called *4-7-8 breathing*, and it operates similarly to box breathing. I find box breathing simpler to master for most people and always teach it first to new clients.

But 4-7-8 breathing has been practiced by yogis and spiritual people for millennia. If something lasts that long, there must be something useful and important about it. In my practice, I teach this technique after box breathing has been mastered, usually on our second meeting. Here's how you do it:

1. **Inhale for four:** Take a slow, deep breath through the nose for a count of four.
2. **Hold for seven:** Gently hold the breath for a count of seven.
3. **Exhale for eight:** As if you had a straw between your lips, exhale slowly for a count of eight.

That's it—now you are operating like a yogi.

What I teach my clients with 4-7-8 breathing is that it can feel challenging to stick to the 4, 7, and 8 of 4-7-8 because some of us have lung capacity larger than others, some of us are more tense than others, or for other reasons.

Beyond that, on some days, 4-7-8 may feel exactly right, and on other days, it may feel too slow or too fast.

I want you to consider 4-7-8 breathing as a flexible exercise. I am not a yogi, and I am not teaching you this technique for any reason other than the calmness it can bring. For that reason, if you find an inhale of 4 to be too brief, try an inhale of 6. If holding for 7 feels too long, try holding for 5. If an exhale of 8 feels too short, try 10! Then try again.

The benefit of the process of finding your best numerical balance is that you will be paying close attention to your breath the entire time you are at it. And attending closely to your breath is breath work at its most basic. You will be winning just by playing around with it.

I had a client who was a swimmer who tried 4-7-8 breathing and found it very effective. But on the day after a big meet, when she was exhausted, she found the rhythm of it too slow. She came in to tell me that her recovery breathing exercise was 6-7-10. She noticed right away that 4-7-8 felt too quick, and she needed to slow down. She tried 5-8-8, then 6-6-9, but eventually settled into 6-7-10. Eventually, she found the longer hold time relaxing and meditative as she took breaks between tasks while catching up on her life the day after an important swim meet.

For me, some days it is 4-7-8. Other days it is 5-6-6. And other days it is 4-6-10. It depends on how depleted or calm I am. Find your own rhythm and know that there isn't a wrong way to practice. It is all just practice, and paying attention to your breath is the practice that brings a centered calmness.

## RECOMMENDATIONS

Here are my recommendations for calming your body:

- **Bronze:** Once or twice a week during the day, practice breath work using box breathing or 4-7-8 breathing. Track your progress by writing down how calm you felt before and after.
- **Silver:** Follow the bronze steps every day and every night as you prepare to sleep.
- **Gold:** Follow the bronze steps at least three times daily. The timing is up to you but do it at different times and use breath work every night when you prepare to sleep. Find your best rhythm and notice how it can change from day to day.

## PREPARE YOUR MIND (BETTER THAN COUNTING SHEEP)

Think of your favorite small child. I'll call mine Madison. Madison is five years old and when she gets bored, she gets frustrated, she may get cranky, and she looks for something to do or someone to do something with. In a five-year-old, it's easy to see that boredom doesn't equal sleepiness. Boredom while not being sleepy leads to . . . boredom. On the other hand, a college student who is bored during a chemistry lecture and happens to be sleepy is going to start doing the head droops and feeling foolish later. Boredom doesn't make anyone sleepy, but boredom can unmask sleepiness.

Bored + not sleepy = bored.

**Bored + sleepy = Zzz.**

The good news is that you have done your body right because you have gotten into bed when you are sleepy. With your box breathing or your 4-7-8 breathing, you've signaled to your brain and body that it can relax, and you are ready to ease into your night of sleep. Next, we will begin to get your mind to fall in line.

Counting sheep is the generations-old technique for drifting off. It always confused me as a kid. What am I doing? I'm counting sheep? Why sheep? Could I count dogs or doughnuts? Mmm. Doughnuts. Okay, doughnuts are a bad idea. But what is with the sheep counting?

If counting sheep works for you, great. Keep counting. I now understand why it works, and I can teach you a new technique that is about five times better.

Counting something, even sheep, is a task for your brain. Sheep are not the most exciting animals—let's face it, we aren't counting mountain lions or dinosaurs here. This technique works because it gives your sleepy brain a counting task, and the task itself is boring. And bored + sleepy = Zzz.

Let's take this up a few notches. Researchers have been studying how we think for more than seventy-five years. Research from George Miller[35] and Nelson Cowan[36] has taught us that most of us hold between four and seven items in our short-term memory at a time. This is why phone numbers are seven digits (before your area code became essential), and social security numbers are nine digits. Short-term memory also replenishes very quickly.

With this information, let's give your brain a task that gives it five things to think about over and over but make them boring. We are going to provide five things because that's easier than seven, and when you have entered the sleepy zone, easier is better. Plus, let's make it something besides sheep. This is called *serial fives*, but let's call it *counting for sleep*, because no one remembers serial fives.

## Counting For Sleep

For this exercise, you need to have a song, phrase, saying, or list that you know by heart. The less you need to think about it the better. If you know all the words or the entire list, it will work. If you were raised in the United States, chances are good that you learned the Pledge of Allegiance in grade school. Here is your chance to put that knowledge to good use in the effort to improve your sleep.

Here are all the instructions:

1. **Say each word in order five time; then move to the next word.**

   It will sound like this in your head:
   I, I, I, I, I
   pledge, pledge, pledge, pledge, pledge
   allegiance, allegiance, allegiance, allegiance, allegiance
   to, to, to, to, to
   the, the, the, the, the
   flag, flag, flag, flag, flag

2. **Continue until the end of the Pledge and begin again at the start. Or maybe switch it up and try the lyrics to your favorite song. I had a client who was a chemist once. He wasn't raised in the US, but he knew the periodic table like the back of his hand:**

   Hydrogen, hydrogen, hydrogen, hydrogen, hydrogen
   Helium, helium, helium, helium, helium
   Lithium, lithium, lithium, lithium, lithium

Want another option? How about making the alphabet a little challenging? Start by repeating the letter *A* five times; then move forward two letters and repeat the letter *D* five times. This option works well for most of my clients:

A, A, A, A, A
B, C
D, D, D, D, D
E, F
G, G, G, G, G
H, I
J, J, J, J, J, J

Try your own list—there is no wrong thing to count for this exercise. Use a prayer, the batting lineup for your favorite World Series baseball team, or the characters in your favorite show.

**3. There is no step three. You have all the instructions.**

Counting for Sleep is useful the first night you use it: It doesn't take practice to make this effective.

Here are my tips for Counting for Sleep:

- **Tip A:** Some of my clients have come back after trying this out and told me they were getting frustrated because they kept losing their place in the Pledge or their song. Here's an insider's tip: Losing track of your train of thought while you are sleepy is a sign that you are getting sleepier. This may seem obvious at first, but when you struggle with sleep every night and you are trying to make some new technique work for you, you may feel frustrated that you aren't performing as well as you think you could. The problem with falling asleep in this scenario is the trying too hard. I

will have tips later for how to disengage from trying to have a perfect night of sleep every night.
- **Tip B:** Remember, bored + sleepy = Zzz. If you complete Counting for Sleep for a few rounds and aren't drifting off, you may not be sleepy right now, but I bet you're bored with the counting thing. The next tip will instruct you on how to handle this.

One final warning—if you are someone who organizes your shoes or the books on your bookshelf by color or the year you bought them, you may find this technique to be invigorating, not boring. You know who you are. And if you don't, you'll figure it out after Counting for Sleep for about ten minutes. If this is you, this technique may keep you awake, not bore you until your sleepiness takes over. I recommend focusing on breathing techniques instead of this one.

## RECOMMENDATIONS

Here are my recommendations for calming your mind:

- **Bronze:** Practice Counting For Sleep when you get into bed each night.
- **Silver:** Practice Counting for Sleep after doing some breath work when you are ready to sleep. Once a week or so, try a different saying, song, or list.
- **Gold:** Practice Counting for Sleep after doing some breath work every night when you are ready to sleep. Every other night, try a different count (e.g., count to seven or count to four) or a different saying, song, or list (e.g., the names of each MLB team, each character on

your favorite show, your favorite song, and so on). Doing this keeps it fresh.

## TIP #6: GET MOVING IMMEDIATELY AFTER YOUR ALARM GOES OFF

You have just finished a night of sleep, and you know it because your alarm has gone off. It's time to get going. You remember tips one and two, and you aren't hitting snooze. That's because you set your alarm to allow you to remain in Disney World (the good sleep) as long as possible, and you know you need to get up now to be on time for the start of your day.

You also remember that you want to get into some daylight by sitting by a window or getting outside or bright light (10,000 lux) as soon as you can to help let your brain know that the day has begun, so it can begin to count down for the night of sleep that is upcoming. Great work, you are already ahead of most people. Now it is time to lean into your chronobiology in another way—encouraging it to work harder for you with something that should come easily for you—eating some breakfast.

I have worked for years with college students. Something has changed for them over the last few decades, in my experience. When I ask about their meals, many more of them now shrug off breakfast than before. They may stop for a coffee or energy drink somewhere, but they aren't eating anything. It's far more common to hear young adults say they eat two meals a day, and breakfast gets skipped. (I'll talk more about caffeine and your chronobiology later.)

Why are they skipping breakfast? When I ask them, they say two things: First, they don't feel hungry at the start of the day. Second, they are already running late and "don't have time to stop and get something." A few of them have a third reason: They are trying to lose weight, and this is the easiest meal to cut out.

If you are working to improve your sleep, I have news for you: You need to eat breakfast after giving your body a chance to wake up. Why? The short answer: Your brain knows you don't eat while you are sleeping but also needs about an hour to get the metabolism going. Your chronobiology looks for eating and drinking as a signal that your day has started.

For the purposes of signaling your brain that you are awake, you don't need to eat much or anything in particular. Any food and drink are helpful.

## RECOMMENDATIONS

Here are my recommendations for waking up and eating:

- **Bronze:** At least three days per week, after about an hour of waking up, eat and drink something. Have something ready to eat that you enjoy.
- **Silver:** Every day, after about an hour of waking up, eat and drink something. Have something ready to eat that you enjoy.
- **Gold:** Every day, eat and drink your healthiest meal of the day for breakfast, sitting near a window or outside.

## TIP #7: BUILD THE SLEEP PRESSURE

Now that your day is underway, it's time to allow your body to develop sleepiness for tonight's sleep. The good news about this tip is you don't have to *do* anything. Much like most of these tips, you simply need to stay out of the way and let your body do what it needs to.

## Sleep Pressure—Sleep's Best Friend

In my work with my insomnia clients, I explain this as *sleep pressure*. Sleep pressure is a simple way of understanding your body's internal system for falling asleep. Throughout the day, every day, your body builds sleep pressure. There is a neurotransmitter called adenosine that helps us relax. First thing in the morning, after a good night of sleep, your body has the least amount of adenosine it will have all day.

The longer you are awake, the stronger the pressure to sleep. Your circadian rhythms are designed to help you operate effectively on a twenty-four-hour cycle. Imagine that hourglass with sand draining again. The sand will drain for fifteen hours (more for some, less for others) starting when you wake up. After the sand drains out entirely, that hourglass will signal to your brain that it's time to settle down for sleep. You might start yawning, stretching, or just thinking that you aren't going to make it another hour before falling asleep. The system works best when you respect it and encourage it (see all the previous tips), and when you have a bad night of sleep, the sleep pressure will return the following night even stronger.

***If it's just about being awake for a long time, why can I easily stay awake late at night when I'm stressed out?***

Under duress, such as an emergency room trip with your son who has broken his wrist on a scooter late on a June night, you can push off the sleep pressure while you focus on helping your son get through the difficult, upsetting, painful situation. You may have been sleepy and drowsy on the couch five minutes before it happened, but for the next six hours, you are awake and capable as a parent. Neurochemically, you have had cortisol overpower your adenosine, and you are awake and capable. When you finally get home at two o'clock in the morning and get your son off to sleep, you go to bed and easily fall into a deep sleep. The pressure was growing throughout the stressful evening, but your brain recognized the situation and helped you push away the fatigue while you dealt with it. Once you were able to settle down, your brain called off the need for alertness. Your sleep pressure was waiting all along and returned in full effect.

The longer you are awake, the more adenosine will build up. This adenosine creates an easy transition to falling asleep and remaining asleep. Adenosine isn't the only reason you fall asleep and stay asleep, but in the neurochemical world, it's a good friend. A lack of adenosine isn't the only reason you feel alert, either, but it does make you feel like doing things other than sleeping.

If you are reading this book, you are probably not having the easiest time with your sleep. Right now, you may be starting to plan a trip to your neurologist to ask them to check your adenosine levels. Set the phone back down and finish reading this. As of the time of my writing this, there is no way to check for adenosine levels. There is also no one developing a measure for your adenosine levels as far as I am aware. For your sake and mine, let's assume your adenosine levels are just fine, okay?

## MAKING GOOD USE OF YOUR ADENOSINE

We are clear now that adenosine is your neurochemical friend, and it will help you sleep. At the end of the day, it will create that sleepy feeling you crave. Here's the thing: Millions of people do something every day that interferes with their adenosine, making the brain's absorption of it uneven and less helpful at bedtime. Are you one of them? In my household, ending this bad habit changed my wife's life, and now she falls asleep easily.

The neurochemical caffeine acts like an impostor in your brain. When your brain sees caffeine coming, it believes it is seeing its old pal adenosine and mistakenly invites the caffeine to visit. Caffeine molecules take the place of adenosine molecules in your brain. Think about that for a minute. Caffeine doesn't give you energy, or wings. Caffeine blocks your natural relaxation neurochemical, and the result is that you *feel* more alert.

What happens when your caffeine wears off? You experience the caffeine crash. Generally, this occurs between four and six hours after you have had your caffeine because that is the half-life of caffeine.

The half-life of caffeine varies due to several things. There are two common ones to be aware of. It's been known for decades that for smokers, it's shorter than four to six hours because nicotine speeds up the rate at which one's body processes caffeine. For women taking oral birth control, it's longer than four to six hours because some of those medications slow the speed at which one's body processes caffeine. (And if you are a smoker who also takes oral birth control, I have no idea how long the half-life is.)

Then there are also the people who love to stop me and tell me that caffeine doesn't affect their sleep: "I'll tell you what, doc. I can drink a cup of coffee and go right to bed and sleep all night."

I love this interaction. It usually goes like this:

> Him [it's nearly always a *him*]: What you are saying doesn't apply to me. I can fall asleep right after I drink coffee.
>
> Me: Some people can. How well do you feel like you are sleeping on those nights?
>
> Him: What? I don't know, but I know I can sleep after I drink caffeine.
>
> Me: Let me ask you this—if my neighbor Tom drank five beers in the last hour, should he drive a car?

Him: No, of course not.

Me: Why not? What wrong with Tom's driving?

Him: The alcohol in the beer is going to make it hard for him to drive safely.

Me: What if Tom told you that he has five beers every night of the week? Would that change your mind?

Him: No. Where are you going with this? This is totally different from me sleeping after coffee.

Me: What if Tom told you that after he drinks five beers, he doesn't feel it? He feels safe to drive because alcohol "doesn't really do anything" to him.

Him: Yeah, but that's just his tolerance to the alcohol.

Me: What does that mean?

Him: He drinks alcohol so much that he doesn't feel it.

Me: Does that mean his driving is safe? That the alcohol has no effect on his brain because he is tolerant to it?

Him: Of course not.

Me: And it's the same with your sleep, only safer. If your body is tolerant to caffeine because you drink it often enough, you won't feel the effects of the caffeine. But your

> sleep will be a mess. It will be less deep and less restful because your brain will be more stimulated and less relaxed. Adenosine, your neurochemical best friend while you are sleeping, will be kept away from your brain for the first four to six hours after you finish drinking your caffeine.

The reasons some people can sleep while caffeinated aren't complicated. First, let's consider tolerance. Most American adults use caffeine daily. But think back to your first cup of coffee or your first Red Bull. Remember that intense energy experience? Remember how revved up you were? How fun that was? Me too. And occasionally, with a very strong cup of coffee, I'll experience that again. Why don't we all get that every time we have caffeine, every day? Same amount of caffeine, diminishing energy. The answer is tolerance. Boo! Tolerance.

Your body comes to expect the caffeine, and you no longer have the same energized experience. Ask a new coffee drinker why they drink it, and they will say, "For the buzz!" Ask a decades-long coffee drinker why they drink it, and they will say, "I like the taste," or "It's part of my routine." The thrill is gone, but the routine remains because the other side of tolerance of caffeine at high-enough levels of use is addiction. Your body expects the caffeine, and without your daily dose, you will have headaches, lower energy, and basically feel like someone threw your ice cream in the dirt.

Here comes the question we started with: If I'm tolerant to the effect of caffeine and I no longer feel the energizing effects of caffeine when I drink it, why not just have a delicious cup of coffee before bed (or an espresso martini or a Red Bull and vodka)? The answer is that the caffeine may no longer make you *feel* alert, but it continues to have the same effect on you, neurochemically.

This works the same way as it did for Tom with his alcohol. He was tolerant to the effects of alcohol but still was pulled over for driving erratically after a typical night at the bar. Just because he didn't *feel* the effects of the alcohol ("I'm fine to drive"), his brain and body still had slowed reaction times due to the impact of alcohol on the brain. It's the same with caffeine—you may not feel the effects anymore, and you may be tired enough to sleep, but your sleep is affected. You won't get the high-quality sleep or restfulness that you would if you finished your caffeine six hours, or even better, ten hours before bedtime.

We aren't done yet, unfortunately. This may seem like a small point, but I want to impress on you how your body works to help you sleep, no matter how you treat it.

Remember that as far as your brain can tell, the caffeine molecule is indistinguishable from the adenosine molecule. Adenosine is a neurochemical that signals the brain to relax. When caffeine molecules enter your brain, they prevent the adenosine from sending its "relax" signal. The longer you are awake, the more adenosine is floating around your brain. This is one of the features of your circadian rhythm system that helps guide your day and your night. Your brain will accept caffeine molecules instead of adenosine molecules because it can't tell them apart. As a result, you will feel less relaxed.

Using your adenosine means allowing your body to get fatigued in the evening. If you'd like to quit using caffeine entirely to allow your body to operate more naturally, I won't stop you. Those I've helped end daily caffeine use have all (yes, 100% of them) been shocked by how *even* their energy felt across the course of the day. Although they all worried they would continue waking up feeling awful until they had their coffee, in reality, they woke up feeling fine once the addiction was ended. And they stopped craving coffee as a pick-me-up later. Quitting caffeine takes a week or two (the first three days are the hardest), and it isn't pleasant, but it also isn't terrible. I won't try talking you into it either, but you won't regret it if you try.

If you plan to continue your caffeine use, let me offer a few tips so that you and your adenosine can remain friends.

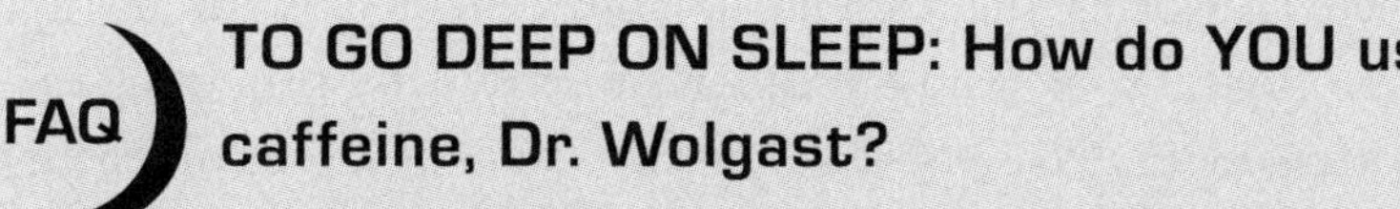


## TO GO DEEP ON SLEEP: How do YOU use caffeine, Dr. Wolgast?

Again, touché.

Caffeine is a neurochemical that can be helpful or harmful, like all the neurochemicals. I like to think of it as a tool. Like all tools it can be used wisely or poorly. Caffeine also comes in delicious and, at times, disgusting packages. (Ever tried caffeinated water?) My goal is to find a delicious path to consume my caffeine (coffee!) and use it at times and in ways that promote alertness when I want it and prevent alertness when I don't want it. Once you understand how caffeine works in your brain and with or against your circadian rhythms, this isn't terribly difficult and can be very enjoyable.

The section in this book about caffeine will tell you everything you need to know to understand how it works and when to use it. So here is my day-to-day outline.

First thing in the morning, I do not drink coffee. I wait until somewhere between 9:00 a.m. and 10:00 a.m. This allows my caffeine to block more adenosine than it would have at 6:30 a.m. When humans start their day, there is very little adenosine in their brains, so coffee (about 150 mg of caffeine) at that time doesn't have as much of an effect on alertness as it does later in the morning.

Then after lunch, usually around 1:00 p.m., I'll have an espresso. Espresso is delicious! Why did it take me so long to discover espresso? I really enjoy this early afternoon treat, and the relatively small amount of caffeine (generally 50–75 mg per serving of espresso) gives me a small boost of alertness at a time of day when my adenosine has grown.

But that's it for the day. No more caffeine. I want to have nine hours for the caffeine to wear off and to allow my adenosine to operate at its full capacity to encourage my sleepiness.

There is evidence that caffeine use, any caffeine use, can disrupt circadian rhythms.[37,38] And I'm sure it's true. When I stop using caffeine for a week or two every year, I quickly notice how even my energy feels across the day. I don't feel the highs and lows that caffeine induces. Eventually, I can't resist the desire for another delicious coffee and I'm back to my routine.

I'm not perfect. But I generally do things better when I understand my limitations. I limit my caffeine intake carefully. I know how much caffeine is contained in what I consume. I avoid caffeine after early afternoon to allow my sleep to be uncaffeinated. And I strive to prolong the days and times when I don't use caffeine. But it is a powerful drug, caffeine, and it comes in such delicious products.

Finally, an important caveat. As you will soon read in the FAQ about drowsy driving, I keep caffeinated gum in my car. And I strongly encourage everyone to do the same because when you have it in your car you don't need to find a store to pull over to buy a coffee or a caffeinated soda when you need it. Caffeine gum doesn't need refrigeration and it doesn't go bad quickly. (It also doesn't taste good, but that's a small price to pay.) I will use caffeinated gum at any time of the day if I am feeling drowsy while driving. Will that have a negative impact on my sleep later that night? Yes. But I'd rather have a mediocre night of sleep than a car accident. And I'd make that choice every time.

## RECOMMENDATIONS

Here are my recommendations for building more sleep pressure:

- **Bronze:** First, finish your caffeine several hours before you intend to go to sleep. Caffeine's half-life is four to six hours, which means that after eight to twelve hours you can feel confident the caffeine is having essentially no impact on you.
    - To take full advantage of your adenosine, finish your last caffeinated item ten to twelve hours before you intend to go to sleep.
    - Bronze medal warm-up period: Finish your last caffeinated item eight to ten hours before you intend to go to sleep.

- **Silver:** Use caffeine more sparingly.
    - Do you drink it three times daily? Try just once or twice. Then just once.
    - Do you drink it every day? Try taking a day off here and there. Then try taking two days off.
    - Do you drink it before and after exercising? Try just before exercise. Then try only before your longest workout of the week.

- **Gold:** Do the bronze and silver recommendations and know what amount of caffeine you are drinking. The FDA and the Mayo Clinic recommend consuming no more than 200–300 mg of caffeine in a two-to-three-hour period and no more than 400 mg per day. Their recommendations are for good heart health, but they are also solid recommendations for everyone.
    - Don't know how much caffeine you are drinking? Most people don't. Use the Caffeine Informer

website (caffeineinformer.com) to get the information you need.

- Here's a helpful fact: Coffee is *unregulated* by the FDA, meaning the amount of caffeine in a "cup" of coffee varies wildly (Caffeineinformer.com can guide you through dozens of common items, from about 75 mg brewed at home to about 350 mg brewed by Starbucks) from one product to another. Most modern-sized cups of coffee are between 100 and 175 mg.
- A "cup" of coffee is not what it used to be. My grandmother's cup of coffee was about eight ounces. The most common "cup" of coffee I see these days is closer to sixteen ounces.
- That means when you see headlines telling you that a "cup" or two of coffee is good for you or bad for you, they are usually referring to an eight-ounce cup, not a Starbucks venti. Scale up for accuracy.
- Here's another: Energy drinks, fitness drinks, soda, and so on *are* regulated by the FDA, and their caffeine amounts remain reliable and consistent.
- If you are trying to decrease your caffeine intake, using regulated caffeinated products is more effective because you can be more confident with the amount of caffeine you are using.

## FAQ TO GO DEEP ON SLEEP: Why is drowsy driving so dangerous?

Drowsy driving is more dangerous than driving under the influence of alcohol. That sounds dramatic, but it's true. Let me explain.

Drowsy driving means feeling very sleepy while operating a car. Drowsy is another word for sleepy. Sleepy is different from tired. Most people I know feel tired at some point every day. Tired, worn out, and fatigued are states that are part emotional, part physical. Feeling drowsy or sleepy means you feel like you could fall asleep easily. Drowsy driving, or sleepy driving, is dangerous because we humans are unable to tell the difference between lightly sleeping and being drowsy but awake.

During my high school years, before my deviated septum was fixed, I was sleeping terribly nightly. I remember frequently fighting sleep while in class. One time, I was drowsy but taking notes and listening to my English teacher, Ms. Bakalar. Ms. Bakalar was a fierce teacher—she was kind, but she was intense. When you showed up, you needed to be on your game. One day, I knew I was headed for a difficult hour because I had been tired all day. After lunch, I was drowsy. I lost my focus on the topic of *Madame Bovary* and had to really fight to make sense of what Ms. Bakalar was saying. I was working hard to make my handwriting look right—it was hard to write regular letters. But at no time did I think I was falling asleep. When class was ending, I wasn't very clear what was talked about, but I was 100% sure I had hidden my sleepiness from my classmates and Ms. Bakalar. Then she walked near my desk and asked me whether I had read the chapter we had been assigned for class today. I assured her I had. She looked directly at me (and I was fully awake now) and said I should finish my reading earlier in the evening so that I could get to bed earlier. "That way you can sleep in a bed, not in a desk," she told me. I remember this exchange as if it happened yesterday.

## MICROSLEEPS

It's no different while driving. The reason I couldn't follow what Ms. Bakalar was talking about is that I was microsleeping. Remember that as a teenager, I was living with obstructive sleep apnea caused by my severely deviated septum. As a result, I was chronically sleep deprived.

Microsleeps are what happen when your brain is desperate for sleep and notices that you seem safe and comfortable. When you are microsleeping, you don't know the difference between being drowsy and being in a microsleep. Microsleeps last for as little as a few seconds and usually happen with your eyes closed—but not always. That means you can look awake to someone in your passenger seat, but your brain is literally asleep. And you don't feel asleep.

When I was twenty years old, I was driving home from my summer job with a friend, Russ, in the passenger seat. It was a ten-hour drive, and I was tired from staying up late the night before, saying goodbye to summer friends. After about an hour of driving, Russ fell asleep, and I was planning to stop somewhere to get a Mountain Dew to help me stay awake. I wasn't exhausted, but I was a bit drowsy. I didn't see any place to buy that Mountain Dew in one town, so I decided we would just keep driving to the next one. We never made it. At some point I had a microsleep and drove off the road. The car flipped, and Russ was unconscious and injured. I was probably asleep for less than ten seconds. But when you're traveling sixty-six miles per hour, not seeing or processing for ten seconds makes safe driving impossible.

Russ recovered and was gracious and understanding about the accident. I felt terrible then, and even as I write this now, thirty-five years later. I still feel the pit in my stomach that has always been there.

My car hit no one else, which was pure luck. Russ and I could have died or had catastrophic injuries due to my microsleep.

The problem with microsleeping when you are driving a car is that you are no longer taking in the information you need to drive safely. When I explain why sleeping while driving is more dangerous than driving while under the influence of alcohol, you'll agree. Driving under the influence of alcohol is very dangerous because your reaction times are slowed, and your decision-making is impaired. Driving while sleeping is more dangerous because you have *no* reaction times and *no* capacity for decision-making at all.

For years now, I have kept caffeinated gum in my car, always. If I feel drowsy while in the car, I know I've got caffeine within reach. I don't need to find a place to stop to buy some; it's just in the car with me. I also know that consumed caffeine (whether in gum or a beverage) needs twenty minutes to be absorbed from my stomach into my bloodstream to begin having an impact on my alertness. So I will find a spot to park the car, close my eyes, and probably nap for fifteen minutes after I've chewed my gum for five minutes. You may have seen me parked in a hotel parking lot or a rest area with my eyes shut, and now you know I'm just waiting for the caffeine to kick in. As a person who used to struggle to stay awake while driving and now understands the danger, this is a must. And caffeinated gum is incredibly cheap compared to the cost and potential pain of the harm that can come from microsleeping while driving.

Let's gather our takeaway points.

**Q: Can you sleep while caffeinated?**

A: Yes.

**Q: Is your sleep worse when you sleep while caffeinated?**

A: Yes. It is less deep and satisfying.

**Q: Most people who can sleep while caffeinated are tolerant to the stimulating effects of caffeine at any time of day, but does this mean their sleep is somehow unaffected by caffeine?**

A: Nope.

**Q: Hey, Wolgast. Caffeine doesn't affect me. How come I can sleep just fine after I drink a Red Bull at 9:00 p.m.?**

A: Just because you have become tolerant to the stimulating effect of caffeine doesn't mean it has no effect. The impact of caffeine on your ability to sleep is similar to the impact of alcohol on how well you drive. Drinking a Red Bull before bed is like drinking beer before taking your driver's test. You can still sleep and drive, but it's not the same.

## TIP #8: NOW THAT YOU'VE BUILT SLEEP PRESSURE, KEEP IT!

You've spent the day building pressure to sleep through all the recommendations above. You've spent time outside, and you've ended caffeine consumption many hours before bedtime. Your circadian rhythms are aligned with your day, your body knows that bedtime is coming, and your body has built sleep pressure through adenosine. Well done! Most of the work is over, but there is a vital aspect to the end of your day that you want to attend to.

Think of the pressure you've built for sleep as putting gas in the tank of your car for a long trip to Sleepytown. You need the gas to start the engine and to power your car for the entire trip. By the end of the day, you've got your car gassed up and ready to go. Sleepytown, here you come!

### Stay awake Until Bedtime (No Nodding Off)

The next challenge is—**stay awake until bedtime**. When the day is ending, most people will spend time watching television or scrolling on their phones or laptops until it's time for bed. If you are a reader, this still applies to you, maybe more so. The problem is, when your brain is tired and bored at the same time, sleepiness shows up powerfully.

### Napping Is the Best

Separate from nodding off, intentional napping is one of the best gifts you can give yourself. Napping boosts your brain power by literally cleaning out some of the natural waste that builds up in your brain. A good metaphor is rebooting your computer: It runs better after rebooting, doesn't it? It's the same for your brain because it allows your brain the chance to "power down" and take care of some of the housecleaning that it likes to do.

Research on napping, or "power naps," from NASA and Harvard researchers clearly shows the cognitive improvement that comes from these brief sleeping experiences. Pilots in a study who used naps increased their alertness by 54% and improved their job performance by 34%.[39] I think we can all agree that improving the job performance of pilots is something to strive for.

The timing and length of your nap will determine whether it will interfere with your night of sleep. Recent research from Melodee Mograss[40] and her team confirmed the general guideline is that an early nap adds to your prior night of sleep, while a late nap borrows from the night to come. Similarly, a short nap, twenty to thirty minutes, allows you to reboot, while a longer nap of beyond an hour and a half can take longer to recover from. You know the feeling—that post-nap grogginess can last hours if you overdo it.

Watching a close game seven of the NBA playoffs or reading a thrilling page-turner means you are unlikely to feel bored, even if you are sleepy. If you are scrolling TikTok or Instagram, your brain is eagerly awaiting the next great blurb to laugh or get upset about. (I'll talk more about your phones and social media later.)

On the other hand, if you are watching episode two of the second season of *The Great British Bake Off* for the third time or reading about how to do meditation, your brain may find some slower moments that unmask your fatigue and sleep pressure.

Call it drifting off, nodding off, dozing off, "resting your eyes for a moment or two," or whatever you like: This is sleeping. Many of my clients tell me about nodding off momentarily and then going to bed later and wondering why they can't fall asleep. Remember how I explained that sleep pressure fuels your tank for your trip to Sleepytown? Well, some cars need a lot of gas just to get the engine started for the trip. And nodding off while watching a rerun of *The Great British Bake Off* could burn up a turbo charge of your gas.

The judges on the show are wondering whether a cake is a good enough "sponge." But your brain has seen this one before, and even though you love watching it again, your brain isn't so curious to see what happens next because it already knows. On top of that, your day was spent without caffeine, and you were outside for ninety minutes walking and talking with a friend. Your body is tired, your circadian rhythms are aligned, and *The Great British Bake Off* reruns are unmasking your sleepiness. Your brain calculates that bored + sleepy = Zzz. And it uses a turbo boost of sleep pressure to get you to nod off.

As far as your brain is concerned, all is well. You've started the sleep car and gotten on the highway to Sleepytown. The problem is, this isn't the right highway: You weren't planning to sleep on your couch all night. Your bed is more comfortable, and you will rest better there if your bed is for sleeping and a good place for you to be. You wake up, probably because your head jerked forward or something on TV alerted you. Unfortunately, you found the first place to pull over on the way to Sleepytown and stopped sleeping when you woke up. Now it's nearly bedtime, but you've already used a big turbo charge of sleep-starter fuel that you no longer have at your disposal.

If you are a great sleeper, or just incredibly sleep deprived, this won't matter much. You'll get up, go to bed, and fall back to sleep. You've maintained the sleepiness and returned to sleep despite getting off the highway for a bit. But if you are a great sleeper, you probably aren't reading this book.

So, if you aren't a great sleeper, you get up from the couch, brush your teeth, and get into bed. Then you try to start the car again and wonder why it was so easy when you weren't trying, and now it's impossible. You can tell you are tired, but just not enough to get started on your trip to Sleepytown. This is the curse of nodding off. The turbo boost of sleep pressure you want to have to start off your night of sleep has been burned up by *The Great British Bake Off* nod-off.

## RECOMMENDATIONS

Here are my recommendations for staying awake until bedtime (no nodding off!):

- **Bronze:** For five nights, pay attention to your alertness across the evenings every night. When do you tend to get sleepy? When do you nod off? Is it a certain time of the evening? Is it during a particular activity? On the sixth night try a new activity at about that time and keep doing something different at that time each night.

- **Silver:** Follow the bronze activities, then add in a light physical activity at the time you generally feel most tired. Walk the dog, walk yourself, put the dishes away, or make your lunch for tomorrow. Feeling less mobile than that? Get a deck of playing cards and play solitaire while standing up at the kitchen counter.
- **Gold:** Follow the silver activities and add a social activity two to three times per week. Call a friend (a phone call, not just texting), take a walk with your partner or neighbor, or go to the grocery store and ask someone for directions or about their day.

## BRINGING IT ALL HOME ON NODDING OFF AND SLEEP PRESSURE

Can you still have a good night of sleep even if you've struggled with nodding off? Sure, you can, but there is some work to do while in bed if you get there and sleep isn't happening. While you are lying in bed feeling frustrated by your lowered sleep pressure due to a nod-off at the hands of a hilarious and cleverly written but previously viewed sitcom, you should get *out of bed* for half an hour and get yourself calm again. Now that you are out of bed, avoid nodding off a second time. (Sleep is for the bed!) And, as I mentioned before, anytime you notice feeling frustrated, annoyed, anxious, or irritated while in bed, it is time to get out of bed to do something else for half an hour. These feelings are counterproductive to sleep, and lying in bed experiencing them only trains your brain to have similar thoughts every time you're in bed.

The reasons you are out of bed while feeling alert, frustrated, annoyed, anxious, or irritated are twofold. First, you are breaking the connection your brain makes between being in bed (your comfy, relaxing, sleepy place) and being annoyed, anxious, or irritated. Remember that your brain and your circadian rhythms are always looking for clues about what is happening and where. Staying in bed while feeling distressed means the next time you get in bed your brain will consider "feeling distressed" as a possible activity while there. Your circadian rhythms will notice how similar the timing is from the night prior and reinforce that "feeling distressed" was what happened last time, so maybe it should feel that way tonight, too.

The second reason you are out of bed while feeling alert, frustrated, annoyed, anxious, or irritated is that you want your sleep pressure to continue to build. Everyone I've spoken to about this, me included, is exceptionally confident that they are not drifting off and waking back up every few seconds or minutes while lying in bed trying to sleep: "I just lie there, looking at the wall and trying to sleep for hours. I remember every minute." The reality is that it is incredibly unlikely, and the confusing part is that you and I can't tell the difference between being awake but lying still in bed and being in stage 1 or light sleep.

The result is that, especially if you are distressed, you can drift back and forth between being awake and light sleep over and over for hours. You won't feel like you are sleeping, and this type of sleep is not the sleep that will restore and refresh you. Stage 1 sleep is built to transition you to deeper sleep—the good stuff. In a sleep lab, we can see this happening, and when we ask the sleeper the next day whether they were awake or drifting in and out of sleep for an hour they will always tell us they were absolutely awake the entire time.

The second reason I'm suggesting getting out of bed when you aren't sleeping is because this ends the drifting off and reawakening cycle that you don't even know is happening. If you can't maintain sleep and you feel distressed, it's time to get out of bed and build back that sleep pressure. If you are a client of mine, you will probably get tired of hearing me say this. This is an incredibly powerful intervention on poor sleep—underestimate it and watch your difficulty sleeping continue. Engage this fully for at least two weeks and watch the changes happen.

Many of my clients will tell me that they can't sleep **at all**. And of course, it is possible. If you are upset enough, you can keep yourself awake for hours. But most of the time, being "awake for hours" is not what is really happening.

Here's the thing: Being awake while lying in bed is boring. Yes, you have things to think about. You have the anxiety and frustration that remind you of the things you didn't accomplish or that you should have done better. And you can dredge up old memories that make you feel sick to your stomach. These can help you stay awake because you are a human. We all have them.

If you are nodding along and saying, "That's me; I am awake doing nothing for hours in bed every night," I have a couple of suggestions for you.

### "I just lie there, looking at the wall and trying to sleep for hours. I remember every minute."

First, I want you to carve out ninety minutes of your day today or tomorrow to sit quietly in a chair with nothing to do: no phone, no laptop, no music, no TV, and no one interrupting you. If you can't do that at home because your kids or pets will be looking for you, go to the public library or somewhere else that provides a place to sit quietly.

Then, I want you to sit there and stay awake. I want you to keep track of your thoughts generally. You don't need to make a checklist of things you thought about but just remember a general overview of the sorts of things that went through your mind. If you are having trouble staying awake, remind yourself of something you wish you hadn't said or done years ago or focus on what you would be doing with your phone if you had it in your hands (but don't get it). These things tend to keep people awake.

Set an alarm for ninety minutes and try not to watch the clock. When the ninety minutes ends, ask yourself how similar that felt to your nighttime experience.

Most of the people I work with find this task impossible. Few are even willing to try it. They say it's too boring or that they couldn't help themselves from falling asleep because there was nothing to do. Also, they tell me it's a waste of time.

I remind them that they are telling me that they do this, usually two to four hours' worth of this, every night. And if they try it out, they will notice that it feels very different, and far more boring, than when they are lying in bed. This is because they are awake the whole time and not drifting in and out of light sleep like they usually are in bed at night. That drifting-off-and-on sleep is neither restorative nor productive, and it steals from your sleep pressure that you effectively built all day.

The other option to test your drifting off in bed is the old pie-pan test. You need two things: a pie pan (aluminum is best) and a big spoon or a butter knife.

Here's how it works: When you fall into light sleep, your muscles relax. If you are holding something, you will likely drop it when you drift into stage 1 sleep. You may have experienced this if you read in bed with an e-book or hold your phone above you while lying in bed. (That can hurt!) Follow these steps to test it for yourself:

- **Step 1:** Place the pie pan upside down next to your bed. You will need to line it up above where your hand will rest on the edge of the bed.
- **Step 2:** Hold the spoon or butter knife in your hand above the pie pan. While you are awake, it will be easy to hold the utensil.
- **Step 3:** When you drift off into stage 1 sleep, you will drop the spoon or knife, and it will land on the pie pan, making a sound that will wake you up.

The first time the noise wakes you up, you will be annoyed and tell yourself you just let it slip. That's because you will feel confident you were still awake. But keep trying this exercise repeatedly. You will have the same experience every time. The spoon will "slip," the noise will rouse you, and you will say, for the tenth time, "I didn't fall asleep; I just let it slip."

See how many times you need to repeat this exercise before you begin to believe that it is impossible for humans to recognize the difference between being quietly awake and being in stage 1 sleep.

## TIP #9: TAKE CONTROL OF YOUR PHONE, YOUR AMAZING PHONE

*If you wanted to invent a device that could rewire our minds, if you wanted to create a society of people who were perpetually distracted, isolated, and overtired, if you wanted to weaken our ability to focus, remember and engage in deep thought, if you wanted to increase our rates of loneliness, anxiety, depression, self-absorption and self-harm, if you wanted to reduce empathy and creativity and encourage polarization and extremism and damage our most important relationships, you'd likely end up with a smartphone.*

**—Catherine Price, How to Break Up With Your Phone: The 30-Day Plan to Take Back Your Life**

As we've already discussed, it wasn't long ago that at around midnight, there was nothing to watch on TV. The networks signed off with the "Star-Spangled Banner," and the next several hours were filled with static or a test signal. (If you don't believe me, ask someone born before 1979. They will remember the days before cable.)

And you remember from my earlier description how, in the mid-1980s, Ted Turner created CNN, the first twenty-four-hour news station, allowing people to catch up on the day's happenings in almost real time. People mocked the idea at the time, but, well, it caught on.

I bring this up again because it's a good place to start the conversation about our phones, social media, and sleep. When CNN was a brand-new, shiny object, many people stayed up late to just watch the news. It was a curiosity, and for some, it became their routine. At the same time, there was a spike in cases of insomnia. The media coined it CNN-insomnia (say it out loud—*CNNinsomnia*—it has a nice ring), and they weren't wrong.

When your brain is trying to power down for the night, as it does every night, what doesn't help is *BREAKING NEWS*. That jolt of adrenaline and cortisol that your body uses to respond to watching a news story about a plane crash, a forest fire, or another school shooting will prevent you from having quality sleep. Even if you can fall asleep, your sleep will be less effective due to the distress your brain experienced processing the twenty-four-hour news cycle while trying to sleep.

The easy remedy in the 1980s was to stop watching CNN at least an hour before bed. Sound familiar? It should. Everyone in my field who's appeared on a talk show or podcast or done a magazine interview has told people to turn their phones off an hour before bed. Why is that?

## THE BLUE LIGHT MISDIRECTION

About the time every teenager and adult in the US started to have their own cellphone, neurologists and sleep specialists like me started warning about the blue light in smartphones (and tablets, laptops, and TVs). Why? Because the blue light emitted from these devices mimics the blue light from the sun: It signals your brain that the sun is still up. Were they right? Yes, it's true, but it's not as powerful as they thought. There is a more insidious reason those devices (especially phones) are challenging your sleep.

First, blue light emitted from your devices does mimic the range of light from the sun that signals to our brains that the sun is up. It is helpful to remove the blue light from your phone, tablet, laptop, and even your TV if you are dedicated. You can usually do this through the settings (on an iPhone, go to *Settings*, then *Display & Brightness*, then *Night Shift*). If you are having difficulty, consider downloading the free software for your phone or tablet called *f.lux (https://justgetflux.com/).* This free download will remove the blue light from your device on the timetable you suggest. Why not set it according to your local sunset?

If you believe you are more sensitive to blue light than most, you could consider buying an inexpensive pair of sunglasses that block blue light. They are often called blue blockers, and they look really, really cool. The kind of glasses people will notice when you go out. The kind that will make people wonder whether they are the glasses your grandfather uses to mow the lawn or that Bono wears to protect his eyes. They are generally made of orangish-yellow lenses. No need to spend much money on these—the cheap ones work as well as the expensive ones.

Another tip with managing the blue light emitted from devices: The farther from your eyes the screen, the less intense the blue light. So your TV gives you less blue light than your laptop, and your laptop/tablet gives you less blue light than your phone. This is because the TV is on the other side of the room, your laptop/tablet is about one to two feet from your face, and your phone is only several inches away.

Why did I call this section "The Blue Light Misdirection"? In magic, the art of misdirection is what often creates the experience of magic. The magician leads us to focus on one thing while the "magic" is happening somewhere else. The misdirection caused by the media's heavy focus on turning off the blue light on phones is that your phone is still very effective at keeping you awake, even without the blue light. You didn't think you'd get off so easily as just downloading an app, turning off your blue light, and then playing games on your phone to get to sleep, did you?

## THE ACTUAL, LARGER PROBLEM

This is also what I call the Amy Schumer problem. A skit of hers took place in a sleep doctor's office, and all the insomnia patients in the waiting room were asked if they were willing to do *anything* to sleep better. Every one of them agreed wholeheartedly. Then they were asked to give up phone usage before bed. They all looked upset and said they couldn't go that far. That is the issue—our phones are designed in such a way that our brains begin to desire them.

Remember the sleep research labs I mentioned earlier that pay regular people without sleep problems to stay awake in their lab for long periods of time to measure how they perform while sleep deprived? They are not allowed caffeine or other substances to stay awake. They can exercise, but no one exercises for eighteen hours. And it's video games that they use to keep them going. As I mentioned earlier, there is nothing more responsive to your input than a well-designed video game. Your brain loves video games because they provide dopamine (the same neurochemical we get from falling in love, having sex, and being intoxicated) when you are playing it.

People who design apps for your phone understand this, too. They design their apps so that you get rewarded with fun, interesting, or exciting moments in an intermittent schedule (so you don't know exactly when it's coming—your brain loves a fun little surprise). This encourages you to stick around a little longer, play one more round, scroll a few more posts, and so on. In other words, the apps on your phone and all social media are explicitly designed to be addictive.

The effect on your alertness from your phone's blue light is mild compared to your brain's dopamine response to games, shopping, pornography, TikTok, Instagram, and texting with a friend.

I regret to inform you that using your phone near bedtime keeps your brain running; it keeps your dopamine pumping—even with the blue light turned off. Don't believe me? Try turning your phone off for one hour before bed and keep track of what you thought about or did. When we get to Camping In, you'll dive deeply into this tip, and it will be hard to deny the difference.

Research from Nicola Hughes and Jolanta Burke[41] and more recently from Rohmotul Islam and their team[42] shows that people who sleep with their phone in another room (like the kitchen) sleep better than people who sleep with their phone in their room. In addition, people who sleep with their phone in their room show this pattern related to effective sleep: A phone in another room is better than a phone in the bedroom turned off, which is better than a phone in the bedroom turned on with the ringer/sound turned off, which is better than a phone in the bedroom turned on. Recommendations for medaling through this technique are at the end of this section.

## START YOUR TECHNOLOGY CURFEW

When I ask people to do this, I get the Amy Schumer reaction most of the time. A few brave souls will take this challenge and try to live without their phones within arm's reach while sleeping. Sounds odd, right? But you know what I'm talking about because you feel similarly. Your brain really, really likes your phone because there is an endless supply of dopamine-pumping material. Your brain loves to feel good, and your phone is the most reliable source of emotional experience you have. Consider trying it for one week. Then, for that week, write down how much you missed out on while the phone was in the other room overnight and how long it took you to catch up on what you missed the next morning. Study that list. Be honest; it's not a long list, is it? Now, decide if you can make it work for another full week without your phone at your bedside.

## MAKE YOUR PHONE LESS THRILLING

Another way to decrease your desire to use your phone near bedtime is to turn on grayscale. I swear it will work for you if you can force yourself to use it.

### How to turn on Grayscale on your iPhone

1. From your iPhone, go to *Settings* > *Accessibility.*
2. Choose *Display & Text Size.*
3. Scroll down and tap *Color Filters.*
4. Turn *Color Filter* on and then choose *Grayscale.* If this feels too dramatic, turn down the color intensity

by half. Your device will now be in black and white or a more washed-out color palette.

5. Additionally, you can also ask Siri to turn on grayscale. Simply enable this by saying, "Hey Siri, turn on Grayscale." Siri will then automatically enable the feature.

Why does this work? Because the beautiful colors of your phone (and especially the way most games on phones use those colors) are exciting to your brain. Your brain gets a little happy (that's dopamine) just looking at the rich, beautiful colors on your phone. When you remove those colors, or even just tone them down by half, your brain is not so thrilled (less dopamine). You can still use your phone without difficulty. You just won't feel as compelled to keep looking at it or using it as you usually are.

Don't believe me? Think you are different? Maybe you are wired to be more rational than the rest of us, right? Prove it to yourself—follow those instructions to turn on grayscale and see how you react. (If the instructions are outdated, simply search the internet for up-to-date instructions that will work for your phone model.)

I'll be honest and admit that among all my recommendations, this one has been most challenging, even for me. I was shocked by how dramatically the appearance of the phone changed and how I felt while I was looking at it in grayscale. I have settled on something in between grayscale and regular color. I can tell the color is washed out, and I notice it isn't as enjoyable to look at, but it's not as challenging as full grayscale.

## RECOMMENDATIONS

Here are my recommendations for reducing your phone's interference with your sleep:

- **Bronze:** Remove the blue light from your screens after sundown (and turn blue light back on with sunrise) with things like f.lux (online, free at https://justgetflux.com/) or a blue-light filter (in your laptop or phone settings). Apple calls theirs *Night Shift.*
- **Silver:** Use the bronze recommendation but also stop using your phone an hour before bed and your laptop or TV forty-five minutes before bed.
- **Gold:** Follow the bronze and silver recommendations. If you are especially sensitive to blue light, or believe yourself to be, get some blue-blocker sunglasses. They aren't expensive, and they will remove all the blue light from your vision. Just don't wear them until after sundown. Remember, blue light during the day is helpful for your sleep at night.
- **Extra credit:** For a weekend, or better yet, for an entire week, end your screen use when the sun goes down or at least three hours before your intended bedtime.

## TEXTING

At the turn of the century, when cell phones were new, the BlackBerry was the hot new phone. It had a full-text keyboard, so it was easy to write emails and direct messages to other BlackBerry owners. (There were no text messages yet.) These were expensive, and people would refer to them as "crackberrys" because they were so addictive.

The addictive part was that you could write a message in text to someone, and they would be able to respond immediately. People got so accustomed to this that they would experience phantom buzzing (feeling an alert when there was no alert) and would constantly check their phones to see if they had new messages.

BlackBerry is still out there, but now all our phones have text messaging. You know how fun it is to be on a rapid-fire string of text messaging with a friend or a group chat: It's practically intoxicating. The fact that a text from a friend can happen out of nowhere at any time of day or night is compelling and exciting. These things pump up your neurochemistry and make you happy in ways that can make it difficult to relax or get to sleep. Not convinced? Ask any teenager with a phone what they most look forward to after lights-out on a Tuesday.

## RECOMMENDATIONS

Here are my recommendations for keeping your texting in check:

- **Bronze:** Stop using your phone forty-five minutes before bed. Turn off your phone's ringer and put it on *do not disturb* until your wake time.
- **Silver:** Turn your phone's ringer off and put the phone in another room for the night.
- **Gold:** Turn your phone off entirely and put it in another room before you get ready for bed.
- **Extra credit:** Spend a week without using your phone after dinner. Let your family and close friends know that you are doing this, so they aren't worried. Turn your phone all the way off after dinner and see what it was like to live back in the old days of the 1990s! If your work won't allow this, maybe you should consider how your work may be impacting your sleep and your health or chat with your boss about whether you can take a few nights off from checking work email to improve your health.

## SOCIAL MEDIA

*And that means that we need to sort of give you a little dopamine hit every once in a while because someone liked or commented on a photo or a post or whatever. And that's going to get you to contribute more content, and that's going to get you more likes and comments. It's a social-validation feedback loop. It's exactly the kind of thing that a hacker like myself would come up with, because you're exploiting a vulnerability in human psychology.*

**Sean Parker, the first president of Facebook, in 2017, explaining how social media, like Facebook, was intentionally designed to keep us engaged**

You've heard the research, and, on some level, you know it's true. Social media isn't healthy for you. Social media is a clever name for something that isn't especially social. It is more like anonymous sharing or gossip among people who don't know one another. What could go wrong with that? If you think that nearly everything could go wrong with that, I agree, and so does all the research I've found.[43,44,45] Additional research is clear: Social media use is especially bad for young teenagers, notably young women, whose experience of self-injury and thoughts of suicide increase as they spend more time with social media platforms.[46,47,48,49,50]

For your sleep, let's consider social media to include everything from Twitter/X, Threads, Reddit, TikTok, Instagram, and Facebook (remember that?) to anything else you might find yourself checking or scrolling through to see updates and humorous or enraging videos. Can you name the most recent social media apps you've looked at? If you are like most Americans, you've checked them in the last two hours or so. If you were born after 2005, it's probably been in the last hour.[51] Am I right?

The issue here is engagement. Your million-year-old brain is designed to process the gossip, funny stories, terrifying tragedies, and so on of about thirty to forty people each day. What Instagram asks your brain to do in twenty minutes of scrolling is to process the highest highs, lowest lows, and weirdest weirds of thousands of people every time you open the app.

One of the reasons people are wistful for the "good ole days" is because life seemed simpler then, which allowed people to generally feel less overwhelmed. There were fewer ways to keep track of people, fewer people to keep track of, and certainly no video evidence of every dropped pot of chili, no graduations filmed from seventeen perspectives, and no immediate notifications when your friend was broken up with.

Our poor brains. They desire to be in the know with gossip and the happenings of the community. But the community our brains were built for evolutionarily was just a few dozen people. Your brain is exhausted by the never-ending stream of input from millions of social media users across the world.

Wait, if my brain is exhausted by social media, why do I feel wide awake after scrolling TikTok for an hour? The answer is how your brain rewards keeping up with the news of the world and gossip. (Your brain experiences social media as gossip, essentially.) The answer is that to reward this sort of information gathering, your brain is bathed in the happy, fun neurochemical dopamine. The scary, anger-tainment sort of scrolling hits different receptors in your brain but makes us even more alert, upset, and less likely to sleep.[52,53]

## RECOMMENDATIONS

Here are my recommendations for keeping your social media use in check:

- **Bronze:** Pick one of your social media apps and delete it. Not all of them, just one. Then see how that feels for a week. What did you miss out on? How bad was that?
- **Silver:** Do the bronze activity and then, with your other social media apps, end your use of them four hours before your intended bedtime.
- **Gold:** Delete all your social media apps for one week. Keep track of how you miss them and how you use your time when you aren't scrolling social media. Consider finding a friend to join you in this effort.
- **Extra credit:** End your social media use entirely and start a new hobby or pledge to spend the time gained on yourself or with a friend or family member you enjoy.

## VIDEO GAMES

We are working our way up the ladder from the least engaging things to do with screens to the most, and here we are at the top of the ladder. Keep in mind the idea that, evolutionarily speaking, your brain isn't much different from those of humans who lived ten thousand or one hundred thousand years ago. And now imagine how their brains would have responded to playing *Call of Duty.* They would be overwhelmed by the graphics and non-stop action. And they would be driven to keep playing it. It's entertaining; it's rewarding their dopamine receptors, making them alert and engaged. Online shopping and pornography aren't quite as engaging, but they are close.

And your brain on *Call of Duty* is the same. It is no accident that games feel "addictive"; your dopamine response in your brain is the same with video games as it is with slot machines. And slot machines are often described as the most behaviorally addictive machines of the last few hundred years.

When people say that they play video games to "relax," they are telling you that they appreciate their dopamine response from playing games. It feels good, but this isn't relaxation. That's because the games are coupled with the heightened level of engagement that comes from playing them. The old parts of our brains are unable to clearly differentiate between real life and the game.

It's easy to imagine *Call of Duty*, *The Legend of Zelda*, and other big system games having this alerting effect. And it's easy to tell your kids or your nephew to get off PlayStation. But before you go lecturing the gamer in your life, remember that the games on your phone that you play work in *just the same way* as far as your brain is concerned. Be honest; you play these games before bedtime, too, don't you? *Candy Crush* on your phone is not the same immersive experience as *Call of Duty* on an eighty-eight-inch television, but *Candy Crush* (or *Royal Match*, *Roblox*, *Age of Empires*, etc.) engages your brain, provides a dopamine rush, and makes it much easier to stay awake longer than you intended.

Are video games the worst thing ever? Of course not. None of the items in this section is inherently bad. Lights, phones, screens, games—all of these things, if used properly, add to your life, communication, and pleasure. Used improperly, they can disrupt your sleep and your circadian rhythms. Remember the Cesar Millan rule—if your dog (or your sleep) is gentle and fun loving, there isn't anything to change. But if your dog (or your sleep) is an aggressive problem, you need to get off your phone.

## RECOMMENDATIONS

Here are my recommendations for keeping your video game use in check:

- **Bronze:** Pick one of your games to get rid of. You can always add it back later, right? Then see how that feels for a week. How much did you miss it?
- **Silver:** Do the bronze activity and then end your use of other games four hours before your intended bedtime.
- **Gold:** Stop playing all your video games (phone and system based) for one week. Keep track of what you miss about playing *and* how you use your time when you aren't killing Bokoblins. Consider finding a friend to join you in this effort.

## TIP #10: MANAGE YOUR MIND AFTER MIDNIGHT

It's two thirty in the morning, and you're awake. You are lying in bed, and your mind is alert and concerned. You woke up thinking about a conversation you had with a friend yesterday. There was that moment when you told them something in a way that didn't come out right, and you could tell they were put off by it. And now it's the middle of the night, and you are awake with nothing else to think about. You are thinking of the many ways you could have said it better—ways that wouldn't have offended them, ways that might have been funny—or maybe you should have just kept your mouth shut and said nothing. Maybe your friend will never talk to you again. Maybe they are telling other people how heartless you are *right now.* Maybe your family will disown you after hearing what you said to your friend.

Has this ever happened to you? Be honest. It has, hasn't it? This is a normal experience for all of us. The middle of the night is a time for reviewing mistakes we made, especially the ones that make us uncomfortable or when we regret what we did. Sure, we can have these thoughts any time of day, but there is something special about the middle of the night that leads to thinking about mistakes, social missteps, and faux pas that is different from the rest of the twenty-four-hour day.

The good news here is that there is a way to extinguish the power of these thoughts in the middle of the night. I'll teach you that after I explain why this happens. The bad news is that there isn't anything we can do to prevent these worry cycles from happening in the middle of the night—it's how we are built as humans. But once you understand why you are having these thoughts, it becomes much easier to put them away and get back to resting, if not sleeping.

Let's start with the explanation. Your body is an amazing thing. It is working all the time to maximize your experience of living through digestion, metabolism, and thinking. That's not to mention the time it spends fighting off viruses, battling infections, and healing bones and injuries. Did you teach it to do all those things? Me neither. And it's amazing.

Your body has also learned how to rest part of the system during quiet times so that it is ready to perform when it is likely to be needed. Your digestive system is primed and ready for food near mealtimes. Remember that hunger pang you got yesterday? That was your digestive system telling you it was ready to eat. Why didn't you get the hunger pang an hour or two earlier? Because that's not the time your body was expecting to have dinner.

The big organs of your body have periods of the day when they are active and periods when they are quiet. They aren't "asleep"; they are just on something like low-power mode—not fully engaged but able to do some of the work if needed. Your body needs organs and systems to have quiet time to rest and be primed for full activity when needed. These times are generally consistent day to day, especially if you keep a consistent schedule, because your brain looks for cues all the time to keep on schedule.

Here's where your brain enters the story. The part of your brain that does the decision-making, planning, and what most of us consider "thinking" is called the frontal lobe. When you are awake, the frontal lobe is busy and active. It makes countless decisions you never even notice, along with the ones you do—*Where should I sit? Chocolate or vanilla? Should I read another page or text my friend? Should I keep trying or break up with them?* It's a busy place. And over millennia, humans have been busiest with thinking during the daylight hours and in the few hours that follow. During those same millennia, humans have mostly been sleeping during the 1:00 a.m. to 5:00 a.m. hours.

What does your brain do as a result? It allows the frontal lobe to go on low-power mode from 1:00 a.m. to 5:00 a.m. This is a quiet time for the part of your brain that does the decision-making and the rational thinking. It makes sense that the time of the twenty-four-hour day when you are most likely asleep, the part of your brain that you need most for decision-making is quietest, right? And let's be honest; most of the time you are asleep between 1:00 a.m. and 5:00 a.m., aren't you? It's just the nights here or there, or maybe a few nights in a row during a particularly bad stretch, when you are awake and thinking about the same problems over and over in the middle of the night.

Here's the other side of the situation: The part of your brain that notices potential threats is on full-power mode in the middle of the night. Being asleep for the last several thousand years was a time when we humans were most vulnerable to attack from animals, storms, and even jealous exes. The amygdala is the part of your brain that operates like an early warning system during the daytime, and it remains active throughout the night because it has been shaped to protect us from threats while we sleep.[54] When we wake in the middle of the night, that fully powered brain system is ready to let us know what it has been noticing—noise, wind, etc.—or it may be replaying the conversation with your friend because of the threat that you have damaged that relationship.

It makes sense, right? When you are awake in the middle of the night, going over and over your mistakes and faux pas, the problem isn't that you forgot to notice these things during the day. The problem is that the part of your brain that would easily manage or deal with these mistakes during the day is on low-power mode while the part of your brain that pays attention to threats (bears and problematic conversations with friends) is fully functioning. Your alerting system is alerting you, and the rational part of your brain is unable to provide the answers or subtle reminders that help you feel grounded. (E.g., "Maybe I did say that today but remember last month when they said the same thing to me? Yeah, I think we've been friends long enough that we will be just fine." That's your frontal lobe.)

Now that you know this, here's how you use this new information: When you awake in the night and begin to get distressed, remind yourself that these thoughts will feel different in just a few hours. Also, ask yourself what is new or useful about your thinking in that moment. Occasionally you will wake with a new idea or a new tactic for how to deal with something or someone. If that is what is happening, get out of bed and write it down! Then get back in bed and remind yourself how awesome you are for coming up with a new idea while sleeping. The brain is amazing, isn't it? Most of the time, however, prepare to talk yourself *out* of going over and over the same upsetting ideas in the middle of the night. Leave a note in the bathroom about your low-power mode brain.

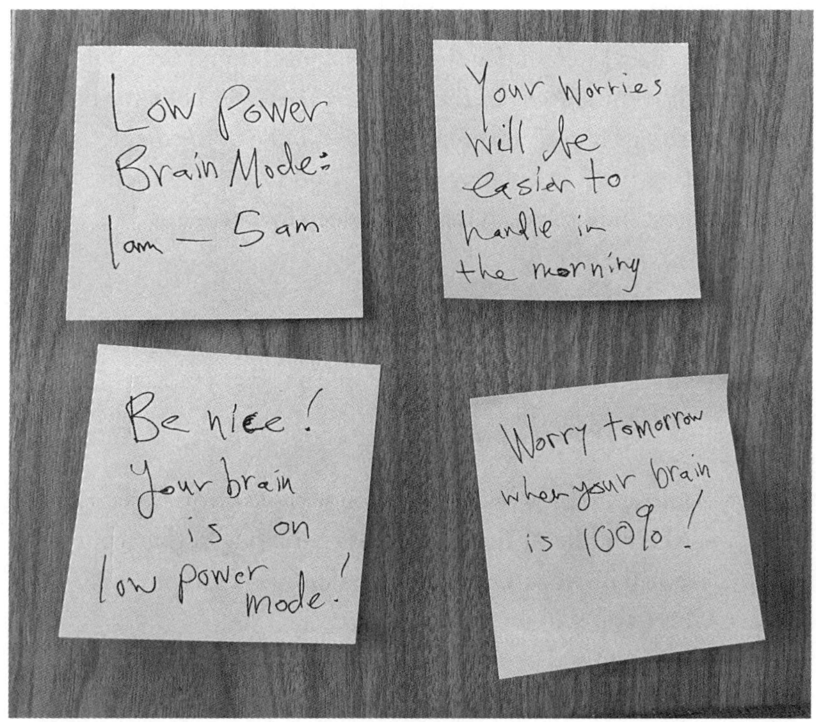


Practice having this conversation with yourself while you are awake: *Hey, self. This thinking at 2:00 a.m. isn't helpful; I'm just revisiting old ideas. I can do better in the morning when I'm not on low-power mode.* Then, have that conversation in your head before you fall asleep at night, so when you wake up, it's easy to remember and refresh.

After talking about this casually over lunch one day, Matt, a coworker, stopped me in the hallway to tell me what a game changer this had been for him. It was such a brief topic at lunch that I hadn't even remembered we had talked about it. A week later, Matt found me and said, "Since we talked about how my brain functions differently in the middle of the night, my sleep has changed drastically. I used to wake up and worry most nights of the week for at least an hour. Now when I wake up with worries, I just remind myself that the worries will feel different in the morning, and I'm built for dealing with these things in the morning, not the middle of the night. 'Nighttime is resting time' is my new mantra, and I can't believe how this simple understanding has changed my sleep for the better."

## RECOMMENDATIONS

Here are my recommendations for managing your mind after midnight:

- **Bronze:** Create a sticky note you will see if you wake up in the middle of the night that reminds you that your brain will work better in a few hours. Place it somewhere you will see if you wake up.
- **Silver:** Move the sticky note each time you "use" the last one. That is, if you wake in the night and are feeling upset, after seeing the note and reminding yourself of its message, your next task is to move the note to a new place where you will also see it. This keeps the note and the message fresher.
- **Gold:** Create a new and even more inspiring sticky note each time you need it. And then find someone to talk to about your frustrating middle-of-the-night experience. It could be your friend, your roommate, a therapist, or someone you meet at the post office—it will probably depend on what your worries were overnight. This will be a chance for you to use your amazing daytime brain

to talk through those worries. Doing this can help you process your nighttime challenges.

## TIP #11: DON'T BELIEVE EVERYTHING YOU THINK

Have you ever been in this situation? You start chatting with someone in a waiting room, or while waiting for something to start, and they mention that they are a great sleeper. You are hungry to learn all the secret tips to their good nights of sleep. You get out your phone to take notes. This is it: You've found someone who has solved the mystery of getting a good night's sleep!

That great sleeper looks at you funny and says, "What do I do for a good night of sleep? I go to bed, and I close my eyes."

You are annoyed. Here is another great sleeper unwilling to share their mysterious sleep secrets.

And maybe that great sleeper can see how frustrated you are, so they tell you, "Well, sometimes I drink some hot tea before bed."

If this is the first time you've had this conversation, you go home and start drinking hot tea before bed. Eventually, you realize that hot tea before bed doesn't put you to sleep.

On the other hand, when I ask my clients who have struggled with insomnia for years, or decades, "What do you need to do to prepare for sleep?" The answers often take a long time to complete. In my practice, I refer to this list as the *Cookie Recipe*. People who experience insomnia may use dozens of items on this list. Usually, they will rotate among them for those with the highest value at any given time.

Ingredients for the Insomnia "Cookie Recipe":

| | |
|---|---|
| hot tea | a snack |
| warm milk | sleep stories |
| exercise close to bedtime | blue-blocker glasses after sundown |
| exercise far from bedtime | red light |
| yoga nidra | deep breathing |
| other yoga | reading |
| hot yoga | sitting in the dark |
| hot bath | walking the dog |
| cold shower | wearing socks to bed |
| white noise | a sleep mask |
| brown noise | ear plugs |
| sounds of the rainforest, rain, ocean, etc. | essential oils |
| the "right" sound machine | candles (the "right" scent) |
| spa music | incense (the "right" scent) |
| a podcast | chanting |
| music | praying |
| a "relaxing" mobile game | a cigarette |
| YouTube videos—just the relaxing ones, I promise | alcohol |
| one or multiple supplements | smoking cannabis |
| one or multiple prescribed sleep medications | CBD oil |
| one or multiple over-the-counter sleep medications | CBD or cannabis gummies |
| a coloring book | the list goes on and on |

Notice that most of the things on this list generally promote sleep. Not all of them (alcohol and cigarettes, I'm looking at you), but nearly all of them. They might be tips that you learned from a great sleeper, TikTok, or your grandmother (but probably not your grandmother's TikTok). The problem poor sleepers have with good tips is that they believe one or many of these things are *vital* to good sleep. The catch is, **the stronger your belief that anything is vital to your sleep, the more you will come to rely on that thing.**

Sleep is not like a cookie recipe where you get the mixture exactly right and always do it the same way. With cookies, when they come out badly, you analyze the process and identify what mistake you made to avoid it the next time. Sleep is more like a crockpot recipe. Sometimes it will come out amazing; and sometimes not so amazing. That doesn't mean you need to change the recipe; just expect it will be good most of the time, but *not all* the time. That's normal. (Thanks for the analogy, Alicia Roth, PhD, DBSM). Let's break down what you *need* for sleep.

W. Chris Winters is a neurologist and a sleep specialist. He is famous for telling people that insomnia hasn't broken their sleep; they were just in the way of their body's natural ability to sleep. He is right. At the end of the day, what we humans need to get sleep is . . . wait for it . . . time passing. Simple, right? It's because sleep is a drive. It's like hunger and thirst—the longer you go without having sleep, nourishment, or water, the stronger your body's drive will grow to get it. Your body will put you to sleep if you wait long enough.

One way insomnia develops out of a problem for a night or two into a chronic issue is through the thoughts people with insomnia start to develop. If you are reading this book, you probably know what yours are off the top of your head. They follow a few common themes and usually begin, "If I don't sleep well tonight . . . "

- I'll be a wreck at work tomorrow.
- I'll fail my exam.

- I'll get fired.
- I'll fall asleep in class/at work.
- I'll develop serious health problems. E.g.,
    - heart disease
    - stroke
    - cancer
    - Alzheimer's
    - early death
- I'll be an emotional wreck.
- I'll be a bad/angry parent/partner/colleague.
- I'll eat unhealthy food.
- I'll fall asleep driving.
- This list could be incredibly long, and we both know it.

My clients all believe some form of these fears, usually one or two devoutly. Ironically, these fears make my clients more distressed. And as we covered earlier, if you are distressed and not dealing with the distress effectively during the day, you will have to deal with it during the time when you have free bandwidth in your thoughts: when you go to bed. As a result, these distressing thoughts become the thing they most despise—reasons to be unable to sleep. It's a perfect feedback loop like a dog chasing its tail: The more one worries about not sleeping, the less likely one will be able to sleep.

Triggering Event
Bad Sleep
"This shouldn't be happening."
"I'll pay more attention when I'm falling asleep."
"I'm more concerned and alert."
"Last night was even worse."
"I'll try harder tonight."
"I knew it. My sleep is broken."

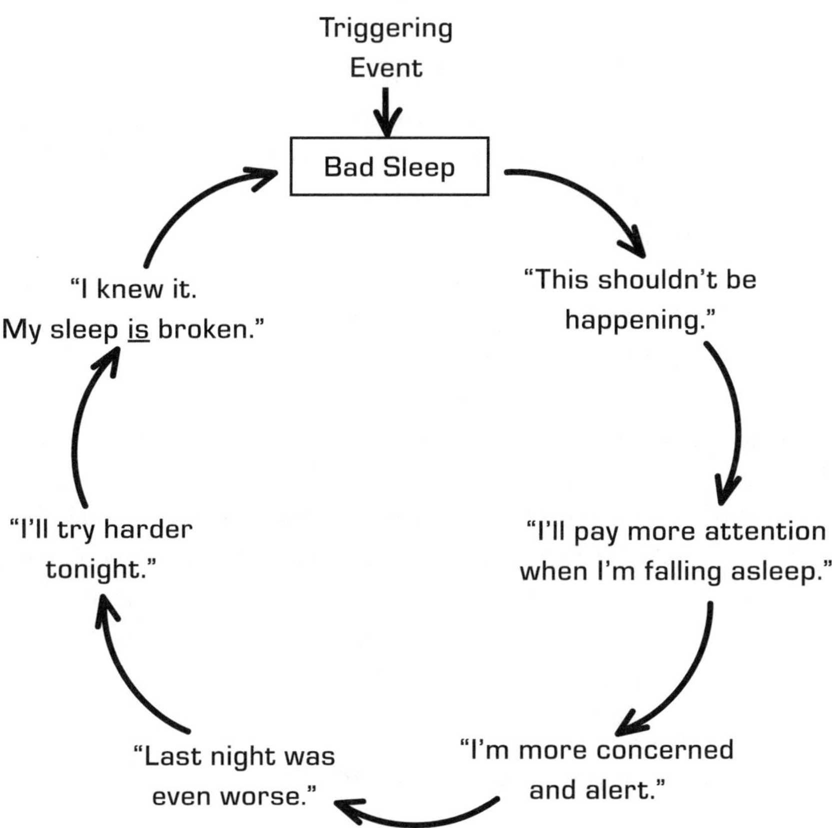

## GOOD NEWS!

If this sounds like you, there is good news for you and for my insomnia clients: These fears are **wrong.** One of the foundations of CBTI is the C: "cognitive," or what you think. When you learn how to fact-check your worried thinking, you can dismiss your unfounded fears and focus on getting to sleep like you want to. This isn't a book for treating insomnia, but let's face it, many people have some misconceptions about how a bad night of sleep will make their lives terrible.

The people I work with have suffered from insomnia for years or decades. When they present me with their list of what will go wrong because they haven't slept, I begin the process of investigating that list with them. This is standard procedure in cognitive and cognitive-behavioral therapy. We investigate things like "How many times have you been fired from your job for being tired?" or "How many car accidents have you had after a night of insomnia?" The answers can be negative and serious, but most of the time the answer is, "Well, not really," "Not yet," or "None, but I'm worried it could happen any day." We take the actual negative experiences seriously and address how to diminish them. Then we spend time learning how to talk back to the unfounded fears that cause enough worry to keep them awake at night.

Sounds easy, right? It's not. These are closely held, personal beliefs that many people have held for years or decades. The more people have looked for problems, the more signs they have found to convince themselves that terrible things are right around the corner if sleep remains terrible.

## THE FOUR HORSEMEN ARTICLES

Another aspect of this challenge is that there are articles that come out every week letting us know that not enough sleep will kill you, give you a stroke or heart attack, make you fat, and so on. I call these "four horsemen" articles and books because they are meant to signal that the end is near—so you'd better get your sleep, or else! And if that doesn't sound like a relaxing way to encourage better sleep to you, I agree.

I encourage my clients, family, and coworkers to take those reports with a grain of salt. Here's the main problem with taking the headlines from massive research about sleep personally: News articles know they don't have your attention for long, so they try to boil things down to quickly digestible nuggets. This means they may not present you with enough information to draw clear conclusions. Here are two ways this brevity leads to misunderstanding the research:

- **The reporting oversimplifies the science.** Research is often reduced to a simple headline that will get the most clicks, but good research rarely can be summarized into blurbs effectively.
  - "Too much sleep will kill you, too!" I've seen this one many times. Yes, people who chronically sleep more than ten hours nightly, for years or decades, have shorter life spans. What is not reported in the article is that those who are sleeping so long for decades usually have medical problems such as chronic illnesses, chronic pain, and so on. Generally, these are people who aren't choosing to have long sleep. If you chronically sleep more than nine hours and don't feel rested, or even if you do, talk about it with a sleep professional.

- **The reporting often leaves out the length of time studied.** Sleep research showing strong correlations between short sleep and major health problems is real, consistent, and convincing. But because reporting often skips over the long timescales involved, many of my new clients arrive worried about their health after reading several "four horsemen" articles, convinced their sleep habits mean disaster is imminent.
  - "Short Sleep causes strokes and dementia!" This is mostly true but not the way most people understand

it. What is missing from this headline is that researchers found this connection when they tracked people *for decades*. This doesn't happen due to one bad night, or even a year of them. This is about a lifetime of bad sleeping.

- "Shift work causes cancer!" For some people who have been doing shift work for decades, there is a correlation with higher rates of cancer. That is true. We need shift workers, and we need to treat them well. One way to treat them well is to encourage them to end their shift work long before retirement. Just like one cigarette doesn't cause lung cancer but many cigarettes make it more likely, one year of shift work won't cause cancer, but decades of shift work seem to make it more likely.

## RECOMMENDATIONS

Here are my recommendations for not believing everything you think:

- **Bronze:** For a week, notice the times you think something about your sleep that worries you and write them down on a piece of paper. Then find time, about fifteen to twenty minutes, hours before bedtime to ask yourself, "What is the evidence for this worry?" and "Are there other ways to explain this worry that I'm not giving enough attention to?"
- **Silver:** Follow those bronze steps and take it further by asking yourself how you would respond if your friend told you this was one of their worries. And then practice

telling them out loud what you would say to them and be kind about it. Stand in front of a mirror and say those things to yourself. "I know that you're worried about everyone thinking you can't do your job because you are tired, but I've got to tell you—no one thinks you are tired. No one has said anything to me about you seeming tired. And I think most people around here are exhausted themselves. At least you are trying to do something about it!"

- **Gold:** This is a two-part process, but you're here for gold, right? First, tell someone you trust about your worries related to sleep. Probably not your boss but a friend, coworker, family member. Ask them what their opinion is about your concerns related to sleep. Listen to their responses and maybe take some notes. Then sit down and write down your worries related to sleep, any other explanations that deserve more attention, and the comments your friend made, and consider what parts of this you can control and what parts you cannot. And work on letting go of those things you cannot control.

## TIP #12: LEARN TO TALK BACK

### Don't Believe Everything You Think: Part II—Common Thoughts That Get in Your Way

If we were playing Family Feud, I would tell you that one hundred of my clients were asked what their most common problematic thoughts around sleep were. The top five answers are on the board. Let's go through them and talk through how to reconsider these worries. Underneath each of the top five answers are several "talk back" thoughts to respond with when you hear these worries come to mind.

1. **If I don't get eight hours of sleep, I'll feel like dog poo tomorrow.**

   This is a very common concern, and while the number of desired sleep hours varies from five to eight or so, the talk-back comments I encourage my clients to use include some clear thinking around the results of limited sleep. First, I encourage them to reflect on their actual experience. Talking back: "Maybe, but remember that you've gotten much less than eight hours before, and you survived." Then, adding to that talking point some details for what didn't happen, "You didn't get fired. You didn't wreck your car. You maintained your life just fine." I also help them acknowledge the reality of fatigue: "It wasn't your best day, but it wasn't your worst." With my clients, I'll know what their sleep is like. But if you are getting less than five and a half hours of sleep night after night, you will certainly feel awful. I suggest you find a CBTI-certified provider or someone with DBSM after their name and get started changing your sleep.

2. **If I have a bad night, I'll be worthless tomorrow.**

   Newsflash: Everyone has a bad night of sleep sometimes. And that's exactly what I encourage my clients to remind themselves. I will also let them know that I sleep badly from time to time, and this is my job. The second talk-back I ask them to use is, "Even sleep experts have bad nights of sleep." And beyond that, I want you to remind yourself that having a bad night of sleep confirms one thing—that you are human. "Having a bad night means I'm normal." The lesson in worrying about your sleep is that worrying about your sleep makes it more likely you will sleep badly. So refocusing the worry can be another talk-back: "My worrying is the problem, not my sleep."

3. **Good sleepers sleep well every night, and that's what I need.**

This seems like more of a wish than a statement of fact when I hear it. People who sleep badly wish there were a simple trick or technique that would move them into the world of being a good sleeper so they never have to think about sleep again. The first talk-back here is similar to the last item: "Having a bad night of sleep means I'm normal because everyone sleeps badly sometimes." The difference is that when a good sleeper has a bad night, they don't dwell on it. They know they will sleep better the following night. And if they don't sleep well the following night, they are certainly going to sleep better the night after that. Talking back about this sounds like, "Good sleepers don't dwell on a bad night, and I won't either. Bad nights are followed by better nights eventually."

People who get in the habit of worrying about their sleep are putting pressure on their sleep. The more pressure you put on your sleep, the more you discourage good sleep because sleep responds to cognitive pressure. Talking back to this idea sounds like, "It's not about tonight's sleep; I need to let my sleep come to me and let go of trying to make it perfect."

4. **If I don't sleep well, I'll develop all the health problems and probably die of all the causes.**

I respect this concern because I know how integral to health and your immune system sleep is. The issue for most people who have this concern is twofold. First, their worries may be interfering with their ability to sleep well, as addressed in the last point. Second, their fears related to their health are usually unrelated to their actual health, which is generally good. People with health problems have their health problems to deal with. People who don't have health problems have more time to worry they will develop health problems.

Talking back about health problems means accepting the reality of sleep and health being tied together but also the reality of how your health is now. "How many health problems have you gotten so far? Let's deal with those first, and then we can deal with your sleep problems alongside them." I like to remind my clients that "most of the people I work with share this sleep fear (some more than others). Most of them have been dealing with poor sleep and insomnia for a decade or more, and almost none of them is dealing with a serious health problem related to not getting enough sleep." Think of sleep's impact on health the same way you think about cigarette smoking or vaping. Quitting smoking begins improving your health that very day. And the longer one goes without smoking the more health improvements there will be. The same goes for improving sleep. Talking back: "I will strive for a healthy relationship with sleep and reap the benefits." For those who *are* dealing with health problems, the goal is to manage your sleep, starting now. Manage the parts of your health issues that you have control over and diminish the impact poor sleep can have on your health. Reading this book is a great start on the sleep journey. Talking back to yourself about your health problem could sound like, "I have _____, but I also have the power to improve my sleep. I'm going to follow Dr. Wolgast's *Gold Medal Sleep* plan as closely as I can."

5. **I will never sleep well again.**

The word I will focus on here is "well" because you will sleep again. What does sleeping well mean to you? Think about it for a few minutes, really. How do you know when you have slept well? Is your goal to sleep a certain number of hours? Is your goal to feel chipper and wide awake all day? Are these goals realistic?

Getting clear on what you are expecting your sleep to do for you is the first step toward removing the pressure around "sleeping well." Get specific about what you are looking for.

Next, remember that as we age, our ability to experience long, uninterrupted deep sleep weakens. It doesn't go away, but it weakens. Don't be angry at your body; be glad you have been allowed to live a long life. Everything becomes less efficient as you age. Sleep is no different.

On the other hand, when you were sixteen years old, you didn't complain that you could no longer sleep like you did when you were in kindergarten, right? You and your body have developed, and that is okay.

On the other side of this coin, even as older adults, we still have good nights of sleep. They just don't resemble the ten-hour nights from our adolescence.

Even those who suffer from insomnia still have some nights of pretty good sleep from time to time.

Be kind to yourself. Your body is doing the best it can with sleep based on what you are providing it. Work on improving your circadian rhythms and your lifestyle and see how much your sleep improves. The fact that you are here, gathering ideas in this book, is a great step.

Remember, your body will get the sleep it needs because sleep is a drive, a nonnegotiable.

## RECOMMENDATIONS

Here are my recommendations for learning to talk back:

- **Bronze:** Review your sleep worries from the last section, "Don't Believe Everything You Think." After a week go back through the list and notice the trend of your concerns: Were they work related? Relationship related? Health/mental health related? Then take stock of the ways you determined to manage those concerns and how many of those worries came true. If you've had more worries not come true than those that did, give yourself a bronze medal.
- **Silver:** Follow the bronze steps and take the additional step of creating a "talk back" comment for each of the items on your list. For instance, if you say to yourself, "If I don't sleep well tonight, I'm going to lose my job," the talk back could be, "I've had bad nights of sleep for

my whole life, and I haven't been fired yet." Develop a talk-back response for each item on the list and practice saying them each time you notice yourself thinking about a worry.

- **Gold:** Follow the silver steps. In addition, select three of your main fears and ask two people in your life how much they notice you struggling with those things from their perspective. For instance, if you worry that you aren't being a good team member at work because you feel exhausted in your afternoon meetings, pick a coworker to talk with about it. Have they ever wondered if you are sleep deprived? Have they noticed a time when your work suffered because you seemed exhausted? It doesn't count if they remember you complaining about poor sleep and feeling exhausted, only if they noticed it on their own. Take notes from this conversation and remind yourself of how effective they found you. Then create sticky notes of the positive takeaways from these conversations and post them on your bathroom mirror or somewhere you are going to see them every morning and night. Each time you look at the mirror, practice saying those top three or four takeaways to yourself out loud.

CHAPTER 4

# PUTTING IT ALL TOGETHER

*Come forth into the light of things, Let Nature be your teacher.*

**William Wordsworth, "The Tables Turned"**

## THE CAMPING SLEEP RESET

Picture this. A bunch of sleep nerds like me get together for a conference every year. We listen to the researchers talk about what is new in our professional world, big ideas, and sometimes new techniques. I regularly attend these meetings. There are always jokes about coffee and who is having too much too late in the day and who couldn't stay awake during the afternoon session. You get it, sleep nerd jokes.

One year, I was chatting with a sleep psychologist after listening to a talk about insomnia treatment. I said to her, "You know what would be faster than all this treatment? Just make our clients go backwoods camping. Then they'd be forced to sleep." We both chuckled because we understood the truth underneath the idea. Take away all the modern conveniences and distractions, be outdoors for all the excellent blue light during the day and the intense darkness after sundown, and voilà! You now have an intensely sleepy person who can't wait to get to bed and whose circadian rhythms are in full effect. And the idea for this book was born. The more I thought about it, the more sense it made.

Since that time, I've tried the Camping Sleep Reset myself at home with my wife. I've refined it and asked a few clients to try it alongside the insomnia treatment we are doing. I've presented it to groups and to Division I athletics teams to maximize performance on game days. I've learned a lot of tricks along the way.

The main concept here is the Camping Sleep Reset. The Camping Sleep Reset leans heavily into rebuilding a strong connection between your daily life and your circadian rhythms. This is done through the choices and behaviors you follow every day. This has to do with limiting screen time and being consistent with your wake times and thoughtful about your caffeine use—all things you have been reading about throughout this book.

There are two main approaches to the Camping Sleep Reset, The Camping Out Sleep Reset (or just Camping Out), and The Camping In Sleep Reset (or Camping In). I'll explain both of these types of Camping Sleep Resets as this section unfolds, but before I get ahead of myself, let me get back to the background on how this became something I strongly believe in.

After that sleep conference when I was back home with my computer and an idea, I dug into the research and found that I wasn't the first to wonder about this idea of camping and sleep. In fact, researchers in Colorado and Japan have tested the theory and found it to be true. In 2017, Ellen Stothard and her team at the University of Colorado took healthy adults camping in the Rocky Mountains in both wintertime and summertime. This was camping without phones, without lighting (other than limited flashlight use), and without screens. A few years later, in 2022, Taisuke Eto and his team in Japan took children camping with a similar "off the grid" style. (Hey researchers—I'm available for your follow-up studies!) Both teams measured all the aspects of sleep and sunlight that I have been writing about. What did they find?

Stothard and her team found that after just a couple of days, the campers' melatonin onset shifted 1.4 hours earlier, making it easier to fall asleep earlier, and they avoided the weekend delay in sleep and wake times that were seen in the control group who didn't camp.[55]

In a second round of Stothard's Colorado study, campers spent a full week outdoors in natural light with no screens or devices. The melatonin onset moved 2.6 hours earlier, and sleep duration increased by 2.3 hours compared to the control group, who remained in their standard environment.[56] That may not sound impressive, but let me tell you, moving melatonin onset AND increasing sleep duration by more than 60 minutes is something every pharmaceutical company has been unable to achieve despite spending billions of dollars on research.[57] Let me say that again in a different way; after a week of camping outdoors with no screens or devices, Stothard's campers experienced improvement to their total sleep time by more than double the amount of the most effective sleep medications available today.[58] These results are powerful and let me know that my hunch was right—camping improves the basics of circadian rhythms and helps sleep be more effective.

These studies measured the amount of light the campers and noncampers received. The hypothesis was that more light outdoors would strengthen circadian rhythms and make sleep easier. They found that campers experienced four times brighter light in summer and thirteen times brighter light in winter camping than their comparison groups at home. These significant differences also account for a boost of melatonin production and realigning of sleep timing with daylight cycles.

One downside of these studies is that there were just a few people involved in each group. The measured outcomes were consistent across participants and seem to be based on basic human physiology, meaning they should be consistent across most people. But it's always great to have a bigger sample, right? Angus Burns, a researcher in Australia, studied the BioBank database of four hundred thousand British people, including their daily activities. Burns found that every hour spent outdoors was associated with fewer insomnia symptoms, easier morning waking, and reduced tiredness.[59] All of these studies underline why more time outdoors would improve sleep and circadian alignment.

In summary, researchers have shown that camping out is great for sleep for the following reasons:

- Bright, natural light during the day strengthens our internal clocks.
- Minimal artificial light in the evening allows for natural melatonin patterns.
- Without screen use or artificial light, weekend sleep maintains consistent patterns, avoiding the Monday morning struggle.
- The physical activity and reduced stress that camping provides result in deeper, longer sleep.

From reading this book, you know everything you need to know to make your sleep healthier and more reliable. You understand why your devices are problematic (not so much the blue light, more the engaging content). You understand why it's an uphill climb to sleep consistently and comfortably. You realize the billion-dollar industries for sleep products and sleep medicines would be happier with you purchasing their products than getting better sleep without their products.

But you also understand how your body works in rhythm with the twenty-four-hour cycle. You know that sleep is a drive that won't be ignored. You know the importance of a consistent wake time. You know all about how powerful the sun is for setting and maintaining your internal circadian rhythms. And you know how putting aside your social media and streaming allows you to power down your mind, let it freewheel, and feel calm. And you know how all these together encourage a better relationship with sleep.

If you put all these things together in one package, you have something that resembles life one hundred years ago, and to some degree, life before the year 2000.

You're reading this and you are getting mad at me, aren't you? You're asking yourself why, if I've had a quick fix for sleep problems from the beginning, are we only talking about it now at the end of the book? "What are you, Wolgast, some sort of jerk?" you're asking your book. No, I'm not. I needed you to understand how we got here, how your body craves sleep, and how your circadian rhythms work in rhythm with the world around you and your daily activities to maintain your day and nights so that this fix makes sense.

Camping out means getting outdoors with little else to do but be outdoors and engage with the natural world. The trouble with camping out is that it isn't sustainable for nearly all of us. We can't camp out year round to maintain our sleep gains. In fact, most of us have trouble carving out a long weekend to camp out, even if we enjoy it. And let's be honest, most people are not backwoods camping enthusiasts. I'm going to dive deeply into the Camping Out Sleep Reset and talk you through how to make camping your sleep's best friend. And then, because most of you will find camping out challenging to fit in your life, I'll describe in detail the Camping *In* Sleep Reset—how to use the camping out principles at home anytime.

## BEFORE WE BEGIN: KEY DEFINITIONS & SCOPE

Before diving into the Camping Sleep Reset, let's clarify a few things: what I mean by camping, what I mean by *quick fix*, what this reset can and cannot fix, and finally, what you can expect in terms of its biggest limitation and biggest gain. Having these definitions up front will help you see the reset for what it is: a tool, not a cure-all.

### What I Mean by Camping

For camping to be your quick sleep reset, it must be the type of camping I'm imagining. This is far from glamping, where you have all the comforts of home, often including Wi-Fi, so you don't miss anything from your social media stream. I mean old-fashioned camping. There should be no electricity, no Wi-Fi, limited access to lighting (I'm picturing a flashlight), and not much else. Am I serious? Yes.

### What I Mean by Quick Fix

The Camping Sleep Reset has provided noticeable improvements in the sleep and circadian rhythms the first night most people use it. However, the more challenges you have day-to-day with your sleep and circadian rhythms, the more time it will take. The people I've worked with have found the best results after two or three nights in a row, and some feel a significant improvement after a full week or even two.

If you are looking to fix your chronic insomnia, I suggest CBTI treatment with someone certified or someone who specializes in treating insomnia. The Camping Sleep Reset may not cure long-standing insomnia, but it's been helpful in breaking some of the most stubborn aspects of insomnia. It's probably helpful to clarify that these were people who already enjoyed camping.

### What This Will (and Won't) Fix

This series of techniques will help address some insomnia (though not all insomnia), unintended delayed sleep phase, jet lag, problems falling asleep, and problems waking too early. It also has the added benefit of assisting with ongoing fatigue, but only if you stick with it long enough. This will not address sleep apnea, narcolepsy, restless limb movement disorder, nightmares, or parasomnias (e.g., sleepwalking, teeth grinding, and REM sleep behavior disorder). Please see your sleep specialist to address these problems and disorders.

### The Biggest Limitation

We can't camp out all the time. This treatment is probably not something you can use tonight or without preparation. Also, when you leave the campsite and go home, you leave the built-in sleep-promoting aspects with it. However, once the Camping Sleep Reset has taken hold, there is nothing stopping you from Camping In at home!

### The Biggest Gain

The reset you gain comes from a strengthening of your circadian rhythms, a reduction in your mental distraction, and an increase in your drive for sleep. Put these together, and what you can experience is a strong drive for sleep, a physical ability to sleep when your body isn't perfectly comfortable, and a circadian rhythm that is heavily wired to the natural rhythms of the day. Let's get started.

## THE CAMPING OUT SLEEP RESET

During college, I worked as a backpacking guide during my summers. After college, one of my first full-time jobs was in the "therapeutic recreation" field, meaning my group would work with about a dozen teenagers for one month at a time. We lived outside in tents and hiked, cooked our own food, and learned how to rely on one another. We had no electronics except for a couple of walkie-talkies that were used about once a day for a few minutes. There were days and nights of high stress, aching muscles and joints, and some injuries. Occasionally, someone would have a poor night of sleep. But in hundreds of days and nights outdoors with hundreds of campers, sleep came to all of us. Although I had no idea at the time, this is where I learned everything I needed to know about the Camping Out Sleep Reset.

The Camping Out Sleep Reset is old-fashioned camping. Getting outside and staying outside for at least a few days and nights away from anything electronic. It works because it strips away modern conveniences, especially artificial light and technology, and allows our brains to rely on the sun and the dark to guide our activities. People who already camp like this understand what I mean, and when I talk with them, they are aware that the Sleep Reset is one of the benefits of camping.

Does that sound simple? It is simple. What I've found challenging is asking people to give up their modern conveniences for more than a few hours, let alone a few days. In this section I'll talk you through how I helped a friend use the Camping Out Sleep Reset to get back in alignment with his circadian rhythms. Once he finishes with the Camping Out Sleep Reset, he begins to use the Camping In Sleep Reset at home. They are both effective by themselves, and they also work well at a team. So, if Camping Out isn't your thing, the next section will be.

### Using the Camping Out Sleep Reset: Lee's Story

Lee came to me after deciding to swallow his pride and ask for sleep advice. Lee and I have known each other for years, but we've never talked about sleep. Mostly, we talk about college basketball and vacation spots. Lee is a successful man in his mid-forties.

He explained that his sleep problems started about three years prior. He knows it started when he was dealing with a big project at work that he oversaw, and a promotion was his if it went well but would go to someone else if it didn't. He began staying up late to get extra work done before bed—first for half an hour, then an hour. His typical bedtime was about 11:00 p.m., but now he was getting into bed at midnight night after night. He also noticed that he needed longer to fall asleep because he would still feel stressed climbing into bed. As the project's deadline drew closer, Lee was working two or three hours beyond his usual bedtime but still getting up at his usual hour to get to work on time. He was now sleeping from about 2:00 a.m. until his standard 6:30 a.m. wake time.

The night after he submitted his project and presented it to his boss and the team, he went out for drinks after work to celebrate because it had gone well, and most of all, he was excited to get his life back. He went to bed that night ready to get some of the sleep back that he lost and was shocked when he couldn't fall asleep. It happens sometimes after he drinks alcohol, but he assumed that after so much missed sleep over the last few weeks he would be out like a light. Instead, he felt ramped up: exhausted but awake. He was awake for hours, and between all the short nights of sleep, the stress, and now the alcohol, he wondered if he had broken something related to his sleep.

The next day, he was exhausted. He went to work and doubled up on coffee. He still struggled to stay awake during some meetings. He also started worrying about getting to sleep that night. *What if I can't sleep again tonight? If I feel this badly today after one bad night of sleep, it's going to be even worse after two nights of terrible sleep.*

You probably know where this story is going. The more Lee worried about sleep during the day, the more trouble he had falling asleep at night. Eventually, going to bed felt stressful because he was confident that he wouldn't sleep well. Unfortunately, this cycle is very effective—worry enough about not sleeping and you will make your worries come true. And the more consistently you complete this cycle, the more likely your nights will become what your body and your mind expect—restlessness and frustration.

Lee fell into a routine of going to bed between 10:00 p.m. and 10:30 p.m. and lying awake until 12:30 a.m. or 1:00 a.m. before drifting off to sleep for five or six hours if he was lucky. He was getting into bed an hour earlier than his typical bedtime because every night he wanted an extra chance to catch up on sleep. Some nights were better, with a quicker time to fall asleep, and he felt like these were "catch-up" nights. Weekends weren't much better, though he was able to sleep in for a few extra hours, and he learned that adding alcohol to his evening made his limited sleep hours feel even less refreshing. While he met most of the criteria for insomnia, he was having enough good nights of sleep to prevent him from receiving a diagnosis.

When he spoke with me, he had "tried it all, and nothing worked." When I asked, he told me that he tried all the techniques for a night or two, but if he didn't find relief quickly, he would drop that technique and move on to the next one. Lee was feeling pressure to improve his sleep because his boss had pulled him aside and let him know that there was a problem. She explained that Lee seemed tired at work, and people were asking her, Lee's boss, if they *had* to meet with Lee for a 3:00 p.m. or 4:00 p.m. meeting since Lee seemed tired and rarely attentive during the late afternoon. It was a shock to Lee. He thought he was fooling everyone at the office. He thought they couldn't tell his lazy afternoons were a drowsy slog until he could leave for the day. After this talk with his boss, he knew that if he didn't clean up his sleep, he could lose the job he worked very hard for and enjoyed.

I know Lee well enough to know when he is worried, and he was worried. I also know him well enough to know he likes a challenge, and as luck would have it, he likes camping out. Lee mentioned that he had a week of vacation time coming that he hadn't decided how to use yet. This is how our conversation went:

Me: Listen, Lee. I've got an idea for you to work on your sleep and use your vacation time doing it. Are you willing to use your vacation week to address your poor sleep habits if it means you would return from vacation with your sleep essentially back on track?

Lee: One week to fix my sleep, and I get to be on vacation? Sounds too good to be true, Wolgast.

[He calls me Wolgast.]

Me: Let me make it sound less good. It would be a week camping without your phone, without a laptop or tablet, without Wi-Fi, and without lights. It would be an unplugged, outdoor experience, sleeping on a sleeping pad or a cot, not a bed. It would mean waking up with the sun each day.

Lee: Okay, that sounds a lot less perfect. Just sounds like camping off the grid, though. How is that supposed to help me?

Me: Read this while you are out there. It explains everything.

*And I hand him the book you're holding.*

Me: Or take another book. Better yet, take anything you are interested in reading or working on—books, magazines, old love letters, crosswords, sudoku, your employee manual. Doesn't matter to me.

In a nutshell, the goal of the Camping Sleep Reset is to do a hard reset on your internal clock. You will be reliant on the sun to guide your activities, not your Outlook calendar. **You will be outdoors all day collecting enough blue light from the sun to overpower your derailed circadian rhythms.** Your brain will feel clearer about when it's time to wake up and when it's time to sleep.

> Lee: That makes sense. So I'll be living like people did one thousand years ago.
>
> Me: Well, that's up to you. I recommend a sleeping bag and a really good sleeping pad or cot for comfort as well as insulation. But if you want to sleep in a bed of hay with animal skins like they did one thousand years ago, it's your party.
>
> Lee: Haha. Your jokes are so fresh. So, once I start, I'll start sleeping better right away, then?
>
> Me: C'mon, Lee. You've been camping before. Have you ever slept well the first night? Even the second night?
>
> Lee: Yeah, no. Never. First night is miserable. Sometimes I can sleep on the second night, but not always.
>
> Me: That's right. There you are without a bed, without a thermostat, without your favorite sheets, comforter, and pillow. You stuff your body in a sleeping bag and can't spread out the way you can in bed. How could you sleep well? This is another layer of the Camping Sleep Reset that works.

Lee: Wait, why does sleeping badly help it work?

Me: Sleeping poorly for some brand-new reasons, like being without a comfortable bed and a too-small cot, makes your body crave sleep even more strongly. Also, when you get back home to your comfy bed, your body will appreciate the improvement and sleep better than before.

Lee: Couldn't I just sleep at home with my thermostat and comfy bed and do this?

Me: You could—that's what I call the *Camping In Reset*, and it's a silver medal for improving your circadian rhythms. But if you want to do as much as you can, as quickly as you can, the Camping Out Sleep Reset is the gold medal.

Lee: I'm here for gold. And the sooner the better. How does camping out work better?

Me: Camping out is closer to living alongside the natural world—the way humans did for thousands of years, until the last several decades. And one thing I can guarantee you is that the Camping Out Sleep Reset will clear away the unhelpful routines and mental clutter that have attached themselves to your healthy sleep drive and allow it to work more effectively.

Lee: You're saying that sleeping like crap in a tent or a cabin will make my internal system want to sleep even more than usual?

Me: Exactly. The more nights of poor sleep you rack up camping, combined with all the nights of poor sleep you've been getting at home, will supercharge your healthy sleep drive. And when it is strong enough to overpower your misaligned circadian rhythms and your fears about not sleeping, the sleep will come.

Lee: My sleep drive is healthy? Even though I can toss and turn for three hours and sleep like crap?

Me: You are getting as much sleep as you need to stay alive. Your sleep drive makes certain of that. You probably get a little more than what you need to stay alive. Eventually, your sleep drive will make sure you sleep. But getting enough sleep to get through your life is not the same as getting enough sleep to live well with a strong immune system and a nicely balanced emotional life with good physical and cognitive skills.

Lee: Okay, so you're telling me that I'll get a terrible night of sleep the first night or two of camping, but that will make my sleep drive stronger for the next night.

Me: It's like you've already read my book. **The more nights of poor sleep you accumulate, the more likely better sleep is going to follow.** This is vital to the whole process. The mantra is "It's not about tonight." That means stop worrying about your sleep tonight—the work you are doing is not about sleeping well tonight. It's about sleeping well in the future. Maybe tomorrow night, maybe in three nights, or maybe further down the road. That's a good reminder not to get too caught up in how badly sleep is going while you are lying awake.

Lee: Got it. I'll sleep badly at first, and that's part of the plan. Eventually, the sleep will come, and I'll be getting awesome sleep!

Me: Let's keep the expectations reasonable. Your poor sleep has been going on for quite a while. You try to sleep for two to three hours without success almost half the nights of the week. You spend your days worrying that your night will be awful. You spend your sleepless hours worrying about how bad your day is going to be tomorrow. Let's set a sleep goal for your *camping out reset* that seems reachable. What seems most important to change for better sleep to you?"

Lee: Gotcha, Wolgast. For me, I want to not lie awake for hours before falling asleep. Maybe just one hour?

Me: I like this as a goal because there are a lot of ways you have control over this. First, you will learn to go to bed when you are sleepy instead of when you are tired or just because it's "bedtime." Then when you are in your sleeping bag, you are going to practice some relaxation and breathing techniques, even though you may not feel what they are doing to help you the first night or the second night. You are going to continue practicing them night after night because you trust me.

Lee: What about that part where I'm supposed to get out of bed if I'm not sleeping?

Me: You'll do that too. After twenty minutes of trying to sleep, you'll get up and out of your tent or cabin and spend thirty minutes looking at the stars or doing some light stretching. Maybe even read a book with your flashlight. Then, it's back to bed with some deep breathing and relaxation exercises.

Lee: But what if I don't fall asleep for hours? Do I just keep repeating this cycle, or do I eventually just lie in the tent?

Me: You keep repeating the cycle, and you **remind yourself that "it's not about tonight," and that the sleep pressure you are building up tonight is going to make it more likely that you sleep better tomorrow night.**

Lee: Right. The sleep pressure. And it builds because my body has a drive to sleep.

Me: You got it. Look how much you know already.

Lee: Okay, so I think I have the idea for how to do nighttime. What about daytime? You started off telling me how this camping would be off the grid. I like to camp, but it's been years since I camped without my phone and some access to the internet.

Me: Don't I know it. You check the college basketball rankings so often, you'd think they change every hour instead of every week.

Lee: I have two words for you: Ken Pom.

Me: Fair enough. For our efforts to change your sleep, the less digital access you have, the better. In fact, the fewer electronic devices you bring along, the better. This aspect of the Camping Sleep Reset is designed to break your brain's habit of having constant updates, constant checking, and infinite content to entertain you. This won't be easy. You and I and everyone else I know are constantly engaged with digital information—some for work, and honestly much more that we choose to engage.

Lee: Like my all-access pass to the NFL Red Zone and NHL All-Access?

Me: Um, yes. One hundred percent. And do you still log on to play *Fortnite* from time to time?

Lee: Well, not like I used to, but I have to stay sharp!

Me: Are you willing to give all of these up for one week?

Lee: If it means my sleep is going to bounce back, I can do that. I'm no Gen Zer. I remember a time when no one had a cell phone or an email address.

Me: It will be like that. It will be like camping used to be before 2000.

Lee: Can I bring a friend? My dog?

Me: Bear can join you. So can your buddy Chimene or a friend if they want. But they have to agree that they will operate under the same guidelines as you. No electronics. No phones. They need to understand that you may be getting up and out of the tent or cabin every night more than once. You may be awake in the nights, and you need them to support that. They must be on board that the true goal of this camping trip is to repair your circadian rhythms.

Lee: You make it sound like a lab experiment. We can also have fun, right?

Me: Well, from my perspective, it's more like a boot camp for your circadian rhythms. But yeah, unlike boot camp, you can have fun during the day and the evening too.

Lee: Come to think of it, I never heard about anyone complaining that they couldn't sleep after a couple of days of boot camp.

Me: Right? With that in mind, you don't have to do army training all day until you drop. But you can take hikes, swim, tell stories, make a campfire, play frisbee golf, surf, canoe, ski, do a ropes course, climb a mountain or a hill, and look for wildlife. I'd prefer if you were out of Wi-Fi range, but I know that's not always easy these days.

Lee: That sounds busy. Do I have to stay active the whole day?

Me: Absolutely not. I encourage you to do something active every day—even just taking a walk is great. But you should also relax—read books, drink tea, write letters to your friends, play card games or board games, plan your next vacation, or do just about anything else you want to.

Lee: Okay, that sounds more like it. Chimene bought a game she really wants to try, and I have this other game I wanted to buy her anyway.

Me: Perfect. Make some plans for what you want to do while you're out there.

Lee: You haven't mentioned my other vices yet, but I'm thinking you aren't going to let me use lots of coffee, alcohol, or even a weed gummy for the weekend. I'm guessing the boot camp aspect of this means that I can't use those things either.

Me: The challenges with alcohol and coffee are that they disrupt your circadian rhythms. Weed gummies? Really?

Lee: I live in Colorado. It's the lifestyle! But I don't need to if it's going to get in the way of what I'm trying to accomplish here. Coffee, that's a different story. I don't know if I can quit coffee for a week.

Me: I hear you. How would it be to finish your coffee before lunch?

Lee: Oh, that's doable. It's not that different from what I do now.

Me: Great—you want about ten hours between your last sip of caffeine and trying to sleep.

Lee: What if I just leave my phone at home?

Me: Now you are on it. What would that be like?

Lee: Um, I haven't been without my phone in arm's reach for years. But I think it would feel kind of good to not have it around.

Me: Perfect. Although depending on how off the grid you go, you may want to have phone access. If you are near a place where people are working or living, check with them that in an emergency you can use their phone and that they will be around while you are out there. If you are truly off the grid (how you define that is up to you), I suggest having a phone nearby that is turned off except in emergencies.

Lee: Fair enough.

Me: Lean into the idea of being away from your devices and make plans for what you'll do each day. As it gets toward dusk, make sure your dinner plans are well underway so that you can be done cleaning up before it's completely dark. No one enjoys cleaning in the dark with a flashlight.

Lee: I know where we will go. There is a cabin in the woods I used to rent. It's five miles off the highway and has running water but no electricity or Wi-Fi. There's a lake for fishing and swimming and lots of trails in the area. I made up a frisbee golf course one time out there. I used to love going there to check out from work—no one can reach me.

Me: Excellent. That sounds perfect. How many days can you commit to being at the cabin?

Lee: I'm serious about kicking this sleep mess I've gotten into. I don't want to lose my job or deal with people who don't want to have meetings with me because I'm sleepy. I'm ready to give it the full week. I'll go from Saturday to Saturday.

Me: And you think Chimene will go with you?

Lee: Bear will for sure. This is his kind of vacation. Chimene probably will for part of it, but I'm not sure she is ready to be off the grid for seven full days.

Me: If it works for her, I suggest she join you at the start and then again at the finish. That will give you someone to share the start of the process, which is going to be accompanied by less sleep, and then a return visit to look forward to from someone who knows where you started the challenge. It's a built-in accountability buddy.

Lee: Sounds great. I bet she will love it.

Me: And if she has to choose between the beginning and the end of the week because her boss is like that, I encourage her to join you at the end of the week. That will give you something to work toward—it's a way to keep you focused on your efforts.

Lee: Cool. I think she will prefer to see me at the end when I'm not as grumpy. Maybe she can even bring me a pizza!

Me: Perfect.

And so, Lee's Camping Out Sleep Reset preparations began. This conversation led to a few others with lots of logistics and ironing out details. About a week before he undertook the Camping Out Sleep Reset, Lee and I talked again.

Lee made the arrangements to rent the cabin miles away from home and distractions. No Wi-Fi or lights but running water, propane for hot water, and a stove. He planned his adventures for each day and included some hiking, reading, crossword puzzles, guitar playing, board games (for when Chimene visits), letter-writing to friends ("I never would have thought of that"), and puzzles. He also created his frisbee golf course, and he even dusted off an old CD player that uses batteries—"You have no idea how hard that was to find"—so that he could have some music with him. He said it was fun finding old CDs to bring along. He brought a flashlight and two lanterns for evening—one battery powered and the other a candle lantern. Neither of these would last more than several hours, and he knew he needed to use them sparingly so they would last throughout the course of the week.

He told me that when he would visit this cabin in years past, he would bring a small generator, about the size of a small suitcase, to power up all kinds of exciting things from home—from his laptop to a TV one year to watch movies on DVD (remember when you could do that?). But this time he would be living without the generator. (He would keep it in his car for an emergency but didn't plan to use it.)

He planned to have coffee in the morning over his stove and maybe one beer at the end of the afternoon (but long before bed). But the plan was to avoid any other substances that would throw off his circadian rhythms.

He was struggling with sleep as much as ever. He was feeling a little bit hopeful and a little bit desperate. This is a good mix for motivation, and I told him so. We talked again just a few days before he left for his Reset:

Lee: I know the first night or two probably won't be great sleep, but how soon can I expect the sleep to come back?

Me: It's going to depend on a lot of things. By the end of the week, you will notice your sleep acting differently, more in line with the sun and night.

Lee: You aren't going to tell me when I'll sleep better, are you?

Me: Nope. I can't. So many things about you and your experiences will determine when things improve.

Lee: And those experiences are mine to choose.

Me: You read my mind.

Lee: Any last-minute tips to promote a faster adjustment to better circadian rhythms and sleep?

Me: Glad you asked. Here are my top tips for your Camping Out Reset trip:

1. **Let the sun shine in!** This Camping Out Sleep Reset works best in a tent, but I know cabins are more comfortable, and that's fine. To maximize the cabin, keep the blinds open or at least partially open while you sleep. In a cabin you won't get much sunlight first

thing unless you let it shine in. And you want as much sunlight streaming in first thing as possible. Gold medal on this? Move your bed/cot to a room that has an east-facing window, even if that's not a bedroom. Make it your bedroom and keep the east-facing window shade open to allow as much sunlight to get to you as early as possible.

2. **No napping during the day.** Get up and keep active. You don't have to be moving all the time but no sitting quietly without anything to do, especially if you are feeling sleepy or after lunch, when it's easiest to nap for a lot of people. Late-day naps steal sleep pressure from your nighttime, and while you are trying to reset, this sort of theft works against all your efforts.
3. **Be outside.** Don't just stay in the cabin—you are out in nature so go outside and be in nature. Come in the cabin for bathroom and water breaks but try to be outdoors as much as possible. You don't have to be in the sunlight, and you don't have to be exercising all day; just being outdoors, even sitting in the shade, will get your circadian rhythms pumping.
4. **Go to bed when you are sleepy,** not just tired. Tired is being worn out or fatigued, and it can help you feel sleepy. But *sleepy* is its own thing: It's the feeling when your eyelids are feeling heavy, your eyes start to water or move slowly, and you know you aren't accomplishing anything (even thinking) anymore. *Sleepy* means it's time for bed.
5. **Enjoy yourself!** This is a week off from work. Yes, you are also trying to rebuild your sleep, but this shouldn't be a week of suffering. When you sleep poorly, just

> think of it as giving yourself more time to enjoy your vacation time. Seriously! Get up, work on a puzzle, play solitaire, doodle, draw, color, or crochet. Or just step outside and look at the stars. If it's cloudy, step outside and see if you can see an owl or other nighttime animals. There are no meetings to prepare for or projects due that you need to focus on. You are on your own time, and if you are awake, enjoy it. And remember, sleep is a drive, and it *will* come back to you.

Lee thanked me and later that week he drove off to the woods with his dog, Bear, and lots of activities to do (some for indoor or rainy days but most for outdoors). He was excited but a bit worried that his sleep problems were going to resist this circadian sleep fix. He also brought a six-pack of beer as his only vice. "That's one beer per night I'm there until Chimene comes up on Friday." He was excited to get back to this cabin and the getaway he had loved but not been to in years.

I met him for lunch on the Monday morning after his week away. He was on his lunch break from work and was ready to tell me all about it.

> Lee: Wolgast, you showed up! Weren't you afraid I'd ambush you and punch you in the face?
>
> Me: Like usual? Yeah, I was ready. The smile on your face told me I would be safe this time.
>
> Lee: So I can't believe I'm saying this, but why doesn't everyone do this to fix their sleep?
>
> Me: It worked, didn't it?

Lee: I have to tell you; I wasn't convinced going in that this would be anything but a week off the grid doing cabin camping. That's not a bad thing for me, and I was looking forward to it. But I did not see how this would be changing my sleep, other than allowing me to get more sleep.

Me: Did you keep your blinds open and sleep in a room with an east-facing window?

Lee: Gold medal me, Wolgast. I did that. I drove to the cabin after work and dinner that Friday, and I was pretty tired. But I figured out which side of the cabin faced east and set my stuff up in the bedroom so that I would face one of those windows. I went to bed and lay there for two hours before falling asleep. And you know what? The sun had other plans for me that weren't sleeping in and catching up on sleep all morning. I was up and cursing you for hours at night and then again for hours my first morning. Do you know how early the sun comes up?

Me: It's pretty early.

Lee: It is. About an hour before I usually wake up. And there was no way I was going to sleep beyond that. *This is my vacation! What are you trying to do to me??* But this was my challenge to myself. So, up I got. I made some breakfast and some coffee—the first and last of the day. Then I went outside and was exhausted. Just wiped. Just cursing you and your Sleep Reset up and down because here I was on my days off, feeling like poop on a stick.

Me: How different is that from how you've been feeling for the last six months?

Lee: Thanks for reminding me. Yeah, so not that different. I got on with my day after a little pity party and hiked slowly around the old places I remember. It was bigger than I remembered it. After all that, I came back and made some lunch and then reset my frisbee golf course and designed the pars for eight holes.

Me: You couldn't find enough trees for nine holes?

Lee: I just got tired after doing eight. It was time to come back and sit down.

Me: Okay, so I want to hear about your second night.

Lee: I bet you do. I was so tired from waking up early and walking around half the day that I barely made it through dinner awake. After I cleaned up the food and put everything away, it was pitch black outside, and I got into bed.

Me: What time was that?

Lee: Probably eight thirty.

Me: When was the last time you went to bed that early?

Lee: When I was in grade school, probably. But also—when was the last time I woke up at sunrise?

Me: Exactly! You were starting to follow the rhythm of the sun after just one day.

Lee: Oh, and aren't you so excited about that?

Me: I'm smiling inside and out. Just to be clear, you said it was pitch black outside at bedtime. What was your lighting situation inside?

Lee: I brought one battery-powered lantern and a bunch of candle lanterns—the kind that make it hard to burn down your cabin. I had a flashlight, too, but that was just for outside.

Me: Perfect. You really did listen to me and my instructions!

Lee: I seriously need this change in my life. So I paid attention.

Me: Great. So, night two you got to bed at eight thirty, then awoke again around sunrise. What time was that?

Lee: I was up and moving around by six thirty in the morning. Lying awake in bed without my phone isn't that interesting. I read a book for ten minutes and then I wanted to get coffee going.

Me: How did that night of sleep feel?

Lee: It was hard sleep—I felt exhausted from the day when I got in bed. Tired muscles. But my mind was relaxed.

Honestly, I noticed how relaxed my mind was and kept thinking how long it had been since I felt that way. It was kind of weird. I told Chimene about it later and said it was like I used to feel when I was a kid.

Me: You mean before cell phones and social media?

Lee: Absolutely. Listen, let me cut to the chase. The rest of the week my sleep remained pretty consistent. I was tired from my days of walking around, playing frisbee golf, reading, and writing letters to friends. I was bored most afternoons, but I wasn't sleepy, which felt weird. I'd eat dinner around six or seven o'clock at night and play solitaire and listen to some music on my CD player. Then by eight thirty or so, I'd be getting ready for bed. When I got in bed, I didn't struggle to fall asleep. I was so tired, and I didn't have anything to worry about—no meetings to wake up for, no worrying, *What if I don't sleep tomorrow? It's going to be terrible.* So sleep showed up, and I went with it.

Me: Why do you think your sleep changed like that?

Lee: I was exhausted by nighttime, even on days when I didn't do much. I was outside most of the days; even the day it rained I sat on the porch of the cabin under the roof and watched the rain. All that time outside and activity made it almost impossible to stay awake at night. I haven't felt like that in a long time.

Me: Did you struggle to sleep any nights other than the first one?

Lee: On Wednesday night or maybe Thursday I woke up after about four hours and was just awake. No reason for it; I didn't even need to pee. I was just awake, and it was about one o'clock in the morning. I stared at the wall for a while, but I didn't freak out because I was already so well rested, and I knew I'd be fine. Also—I didn't have anything I needed to be sharp for the next day. So I was awake for half an hour, maybe forty-five minutes, and I just did some deep breathing like you taught me. The next thing I knew the sun was busting through the windows, and it was hours later.

Me: Sounds like by Wednesday you had caught up on sleep and didn't get worried about being awake, so you eventually went back to sleep. I'll let you in on a secret about that.

Lee: What is it?

Me: That's how people who sleep well go through a random awakening in the night. It happens, but it doesn't worry them. They know they'll get back to sleep and be fine the next day.

Lee: Well, dang. And that was me!

Me: You have come out on the other side of your sleep problems. Did Chimene come to visit?

Lee: She came on Friday—left work at noon, and we spent most of Friday and Saturday up there. She brought a pizza from the town nearby and a couple of beers for me. It was fun showing her around and having someone to talk to. I did meet some people while I was out there who were also hiking and staying in cabins, but it was great to have Chimene with me.

Me: Lots of times, when you meet other people camping, they invite you to hang out in the evening, eat food, or share some dessert or a drink. Did that happen?

Lee: I got invited to hang out by one group, but I think most people aren't excited to invite a single man and his dog to hang out in the evening while camping in the middle of nowhere. So I visited that group for a bit before dinner, and we ate together and played cards on the last night they were there. But I got back to my cabin by eight o'clock at night, and I didn't drink any alcohol with them. They were really interested in my Camping Sleep Reset experience.

Me: Really? What did they say?

Lee: After I told them about it, they thought it was so obvious that camping and improving sleep go hand in hand. They camp a lot, and they were talking about how they never thought about it before, but they always go home feeling not only happy to sleep in their beds again but also rested in more than just a physical way.

Me: That raises the question—what was it like for you when you got home? Back to reality and all the electronics.

Lee: Well, I talked about it a lot when Chimene came up to visit and had obviously been thinking about the experience for days. I decided I would try to maintain what I gained when I got home with some of what I learned. First, I decided to turn off the TV and put my phone away ninety minutes before bed.

Me: If I asked you to do that a month ago, what would you have said?

Lee: I would have been polite about it, but I would have told you where you could stick that idea.

Me: So what about this experience changed your mind?

Lee: After the Camping Out Reset, I felt more relaxed and clearheaded in the evenings than I have for years. Honestly, I don't know how long it's been since I felt that clear. It was amazing. I wanted to hang on to that feeling, and turning off the TV and my phone seemed like a very reasonable thing to do.

Me: I love it. Glad you got to that. What else did you do to your daily routine now that you are back at home?

Lee: I open my blinds immediately after I get out of bed. I sit near the window, any window, all the time. I spend time outside during lunch instead of sitting at my desk. After work, I walk the long route to my car, so I can spend more time outside. All in all, it's not like camping, but I'm getting about two hours more sunlight every day than I used to.

Me: I wish everyone would do that. It's so much better for you and your overall health.

Lee: I still can't believe this worked. I don't get eight or nine hours of sleep every night; I probably get more like seven or eight on the weekends. But the biggest difference is that I know I will get to sleep and be okay. I know it took a week of my vacation time and a lot of effort, but in the end, it was simple. I just needed to live like someone who doesn't live in the twenty-first century.

Me: I'm super happy to hear this. What's it like at work?

Lee: As soon as I got back, two people told me I must have had a great vacation because I seemed so relaxed. I told my boss the whole story, and she went from thinking it was a stupid idea to being convinced. She told me she is thinking of telling her husband they should try something like that. I'm going to loan them your book.

Me: Outstanding. I couldn't be happier for you. Keep up the good work and remember those main principles when you have a rough night or two or a stressful week at work. You can do this—there wasn't anything out at that cabin that you can't recreate in your life. Well, the quiet and the space isn't your everyday, but you know what I mean.

Lee: Thanks, Wolgast. I feel like I have my life back, and I definitely have my job back.

Wait, I Hate Camping! What Can I Do for a Quick Fix??

## THE CAMPING IN SLEEP RESET—SILVER AND BRONZE

When I talk to people about the Camping Out Sleep Reset, they generally have one of two reactions. The first, which comes from a much smaller group, gets excited and starts digging out their old tent. They are ready to double down and grab the gold medal with a camping trip. But the much larger group will tell me that it sounds like a good idea, but they "seriously hate camping."

When I met my wife, one of the things we talked about was my love of the outdoors. She shares that, and we have had many adventures together, even hiked a few fourteeners in Colorado with the kids. She is not afraid of the outdoors and loves the thrill of getting out there to enjoy it. But from the start, she made one thing clear: "If you are camping out, you can have fun with your friends and meet me at the hotel when you're done." Loud and clear. She doesn't sleep outdoors. We made our peace around this and have had a great time finding outdoor activities we both love.

If you reread the Camping Out Sleep Reset section, you'll notice that the main factors I lean into don't have much to do with camping itself—the focus is on aligning your circadian rhythms with the natural rhythms of the world around you by avoiding the aspects of our daily lives that go against the grain of those natural rhythms.

Camping out isn't essential to do that; it just does the work for you. There is little to think about with camping when you're trying to reset your circadian rhythms because you are taking yourself back to the way things worked for the three hundred thousand years before we got electricity, Wi-Fi, and TikTok.

While the Camping Out Reset has some research to support it, the Camping In Reset does not. The Camping In Reset is based on the lessons of circadian rhythm science and the research from the Camping Out Reset. The ideas of Camping In Reset are half steps away from the research that supports the Camping Out Reset.[60] For me, that's more than enough. But if you are a researcher and would like to partner with me to study The Camping In Reset, I am available and excited to hear from you. If you are not a researcher, but you want to tell me about your experience trying out the Camping In Reset, find my website GoldMedalSleep.com and do it! I love hearing and sharing how people have reacted to this experience. You can also share your ideas with me there that I can promote when I talk to new people about this and when I write the follow up to this book.

The biggest differences between Camping Out and Camping In have to do with you controlling your morning wake up and your evening wind down. Rather than watching the sun go down over the hill or mountain, you will be acting like the power is out at home. Rather than spending your days outdoors walking or relaxing, you'll be doing your regular routine of work or school and finding windows for sunlight and windows of time when you can be outdoors. And most challenging for most people, you'll be in charge of ending your electronic and phone use hours before bedtime. Can you reset your circadian rhythms without camping outside? You certainly can. Let's talk about how to do the **Camping In Sleep Reset** at home!

## Camping In with Alex

I briefly introduced you to Alex in the introduction to this book, but let's get to know her better now. Alex saw me speak at her college and came up to me afterward to introduce herself and tell me that she wished she had met me as a sophomore when she was struggling with insomnia, which had since improved.

Alex contacted me a few years later as a twenty-four-year-old, first-year medical student, worried that her old insomnia was returning. I felt like I knew her well after an hour of talking through her issues. Alex is an intense young woman. Bright, funny, and direct. Growing up, she was an intimidating soccer midfielder on a national league contender ("We sort of won nationals the year of COVID because we were the only team who qualified before the world shut down") but made the choice in college to forgo her athletics for academics. She wanted to be a doctor after her dad had fought off a brutal cancer.

In college, she had developed insomnia at a time when her schedule was erratic (waking at 8:00 a.m. on Mondays, Wednesdays, and Fridays; then at 10:30 a.m. on Tuesdays and Thursdays; and then at noon or 1:00 p.m. on Saturdays and Sundays). While her sleep/wake schedule was erratic by most standards, it was normal for a college student.

During her sophomore year she was involved in a bad car accident. Alex had minor injuries from the accident but felt on edge for weeks afterward, making sleep difficult—it would take her from one to two hours to fall asleep, and usually she would wake up an hour before her alarm was set to go off, feeling wide awake. Then she began to worry that she had lost her ability to fall asleep. She struggled with insomnia every night of the week for two years. It took her nearly two more years of trying different things, but over one summer break from college, she got back on a regular schedule and was able to sleep consistently and reliably again. She grew confident about her sleep, her insomnia was gone, and she was pleased to be back to her normal life. Her takeaway from this experience was that she never wanted to go through that again.

Starting medical school with all it demands from her time, she worried that her old insomnia was creeping back in, an insomnia she thought she had gotten rid of three years before.

Classes had begun, and she was struggling to sleep at night. A few nights per week, it could take her an hour or more to fall asleep. Once she got to sleep, the nights usually went smoothly with no interruptions to her sleep—she slept well until about an hour before her alarm. Combining the trouble she had at the start of her nights, she had about an hour of insomnia when she would wake up too early two to three nights per week. "It's not as bad as when I was in college, but it's starting to feel like I could slide back to that bad insomnia. I got worried and called you," she said.

Her ability to study and focus during her classes was compromised. When she came to me, she said, "I didn't work my ass off in high school and college for the last eight years to fall apart now that medical school has started. I've got to get back to sleeping on my own. I have to make this work."

I learned about her previous insomnia history and how it took a summer internship with a regular 9:00 a.m. start time to get her back on track. Alex also told me that she doesn't take any medications, rarely drinks alcohol, and avoids cannabis and other substances "to stay sharp." The car accident that was the starting gun for her previous insomnia was years in the past, and it wasn't bothering her now. She hadn't had a nightmare in over a year. But she was struggling to stay awake every day during classes and would usually get a burst of energy late in the evening, around 11:00 p.m., which made it difficult for her to fall asleep when she wanted. Her preferred bedtime was about midnight, and she wished she could wake up at 7:00 a.m., but often was wide awake in bed at 6:00 a.m. This had been going on for about three straight weeks, three or four nights per week. She cured her insomnia that first time by maintaining a consistent, relaxed schedule for one entire summer, and this time around, she didn't have that time or relaxed schedule.

We discussed how what she was experiencing hadn't gone on long enough to constitute an insomnia diagnosis, but it wasn't too soon to start working her way out of it. We discussed the standard insomnia treatment for stubborn insomnia—CBTI, and its standard six-to-ten-week treatment course. Alex was disappointed to hear about how long that would take:

> Alex: I don't think I have the time for that to take effect. I mean, eight weeks from now midterm exams will already be over, and I need to catch up already. Maybe I just need to ask my doctor for a medication to get me through.
>
> Me: You could talk to your doctor about medications, but you've already told me that you want to avoid medication for sleep since you know sleep is something you used to do without a problem on your own. There is another technique that is based on your circadian rhythms, and it's worked for some of my dedicated clients, but while the research is promising, it was done with only a couple dozen people.
>
> Alex: I'm listening.
>
> Me: The technique of the Camping Out Sleep Reset supercharges your circadian rhythms, and it was built for people who could take time away from work or school to get out camping.
>
> Alex: Um, yeah. Not sure my professors are going to be interested in that.

Me: Right—bear with me. That technique is like the gold medal; you go camping for a week and follow my instructions. But if you are willing to aim for a silver or bronze medal, there are ways to do most of this while you are living your life as a medical student. It's called the Camping In Sleep Reset, and it makes for a strong reset on your sleep in about two weeks.

Alex: Gold is overrated. Any medal is better than where my sleep is heading right now.

Me: I couldn't agree more. My sense is that you have good sleep when you actually do sleep, but you have several systems internally that you have trained to work against sleep for the last few years. You need to retrain your brain to pay close attention to the world around you so that sleep becomes part of the daily routines.

Alex: Um, that sounds too simple. I am sleeping badly. Convince me this will work.

Me: I hear you. The process is going to be hard. I'm going to ask you to change your lifestyle quite a bit for two weeks. You'll need to do most of, or better yet, all your studying before the sun goes down. You'll need to be sure to get outside every day for at least thirty minutes, though several hours of outdoor time is better. You'll also need a blue light to work with.

Alex: I usually finish studying later in the night, then I take a shower and go to bed. Not sure I can get all the studying done before the sun goes down. Last night it was getting dark at eight o'clock.

Me: And the later you go into the semester, the earlier the sun will go down. For now, you have the September sunset at your guidepost.

Alex: But how is this supposed to help me? I don't get it.

Me: We are going to keep you in the daytime world of a busy medical student in Philadelphia, but we are going to reintroduce your circadian rhythms to the old-world evenings and nighttime—before cell phones, computers, and electricity. This may not sound like much because we are all so accustomed to the modern world. But your brain is going to react in ways you probably haven't experienced since you were a little kid. You will feel sleepier earlier and more relaxed waking up.

Alex: I'm going to call myself skeptical, but I'm interested because it sounds like you are describing using my body and my brain to fix my sleep, not medication or some sleep product.

Me: We are on the same page now. There is only one thing I'd like you to purchase, and you can find one for under thirty dollars—it's a blue light lamp. You'll need this to strengthen your morning waking experience since medical school has you spending most of the rest of your day inside and not near windows.

Alex: I can do that. I think my sister has one of those I can use.

Me: That's fine; just make sure it will produce 10,000 lux of light so that we know it's doing what we want it to do for you.

Alex: Okay, what's the rest of the process?

Me: Let's start first thing in the morning and work our way through the day, okay?

Alex: Sure.

Me: Camping In is a two-week process. I can promise you that after the first week your sleep will feel different to you, but you need to maintain these strategies for two straight weeks for them to become sticky, like a habit. Can you commit to two weeks?

Alex: I am willing to consider it, but I need to know what you are asking first.

Me: Fair enough. Let's go through the steps. You want to wake up at 7:00 a.m., right?

## Camping In Reset Starts When the Day Starts

The Camping In Reset will start to feel like it is heavily focused on your evenings and bedtime. But it won't work as well if you don't change your mornings. Mornings are when you reset your biggest circadian clock timers with sunlight. Taking advantage of this massive influence on your circadian rhythm gets you started on the right foot for the entire day. Getting early morning blue light, especially sunlight, followed by more sunlight throughout the day, makes your evenings and bedtime much easier.[61,62] This is backed up with consistent data from the scientific worlds of physiology and circadian science.

A video game analogy helps some of the people I've worked with to understand this concept. Using the sun first thing in the morning is like getting two power-ups or buying several advantages in a video game. It can make the difference between needing nearly perfect game play to succeed compared to just easing your way into the finish. Much of the work is done for you by the sunlight, and the more bright light across the day, the more the advantage is for you.

> Alex: Right.
>
> Me: Keep your alarm set for 7:00 a.m. and maintain that wake-up time every day. Even on weekends.
>
> Alex: Ugh. Ouch. Weekdays, I wake up earlier than that, which annoys me. But weekends, I usually sleep in. Just for two weeks, right?
>
> Me: Right, not forever. But the minor pain has only just begun. This is the first step to rebuilding your circadian rhythms. Also, you will have left the window blinds up at bedtime, so most of the window will let sunshine in. That will help you feel like it's time to wake up.
>
> Alex: I thought sleep doctors are always telling everyone to have blackout curtains and a pitch-black bedroom. What is this about?
>
> Me: I'm not trying to get you to sleep deeply; we are trying to reset your circadian rhythms. The sunlight is your most

powerful friend in this process. You need to welcome it every day. Deep sleep will follow when strong circadian rhythms are in place.

Alex: My window is right next to a streetlight outside. If I leave my blinds open, it will be shining in my room all night.

Me: That's a shame. Then for you, I want you to open your blind immediately when you wake up. You need to get that early morning light in your room. When the alarm goes off, you are up and out of bed within a minute or two—no snoozing.

Alex: I'm usually awake earlier than that because I can't sleep, so I can do that.

Me: Great. Well, not great you aren't sleeping, but great you can get moving. Once you are up, you need to get even more blue light, especially if your window doesn't face east. What is your morning routine like?

Alex: I don't really eat breakfast or anything; I just wash my face, brush my teeth, get dressed, and grab snacks for later.

Me: Your body needs about an hour to get its metabolism going, so you can wait a bit to eat and drink something. But then it's important to get something in your body—food and drink. You can drink water immediately and even black coffee. But an hour after you wake up, eat something.

## CONSISTENT MEAL TIMING MAINTAINS CIRCADIAN RHYTHMS, TOO

Accordiong to Laura Pickel and Hoon-Ki Sung, while light is the main cue for our central internal clocks, meal timing is the dominant cue for peripheral clocks.[63] Researchers like Shubhroz Gill[64] and Yu Tahara,[65] who study circadian rhythms and nutrition, have been telling us for years that the timing of our meals is another aspect of daily living that helps regulate our internal clocks. When we eat at consistent times, our bodies operate better and are clearer about when it is time to be awake and be asleep.

Turns out that the timing of our meals and snacks is information used by our circadian rhythms too. It shouldn't surprise you this late in my book that our bodies are looking for information about what they should be doing at a particular time of day and using things like meals and nutrition input as data.

I may sound like your grandmother in telling you this, but the recommendations are to

- eat your meals at roughly the same time every day,
- avoid late-night eating or snacking, and
- finish eating for the day at least two hours before your planned bedtime; more hours before bedtime is better.

Alex: Does it matter what I eat?

Me: It doesn't have to be much; just something in your belly to let your body know that you have started your day. Healthier food leads to healthier sleep; so think of it that way. Could be two bites of a banana, a few nuts, a piece of a bagel, or a full breakfast—anything. And something to drink—a glass of water is fine, but I'm going to guess that you have coffee soon after you wake up.

Alex: Yep. I make my coffee to take with me on my way to classes.

Me: In that case, find a snack or two at the grocery store to go along with your coffee and make it easy to take with you. Buy enough ahead of time so that you can have a snack every day for two weeks.

Alex: Got it. Buy snacks to take with me—eat them an hour after I wake up.

Me: Then, you need to decide where you are going to have your blue light placed so that it does its work. I'd like for you to have twenty minutes of time where the blue light is on and in your field of vision.

Alex: I can put it on the sink while I'm getting ready.

Me: Great. You don't need to look at the blue light—you just need it to be somewhere your eyes see it. The sink should be fine. Then, keep an eye on how long it takes you in the bathroom to get ready. If it's not a full twenty minutes, just bring the blue light with you from the bathroom to your bedroom while you are getting dressed. Once you've hit that twenty-minute mark, you can turn it off until you wake up the next day. They do make some nice blue-light glasses you can just wear for twenty minutes, but they are much more expensive.

Alex: Yeah, I'd rather borrow my sister's blue light for free. Okay, I'm up at 7:00 a.m. and moving, and I get twenty minutes of blue light while I get ready. An hour later I eat and drink something. Then what?

Me: I'd like you to get outside between classes to maximize your access to sunlight. If it's raining, just get to a big window and sit nearby facing the window.

Alex: Do I have to stare out the window like a complete idiot?

Me: Do what you want to do—you can even check Instagram while you are there. If you can eat lunch outside, even better. Better yet, take a walk outside.

Alex: This all sounds kind of normal.

Me: It is, but I'm going to guess that you don't eat lunch near a window every day, nor do you take a walk during the day every day.

Alex: Nope. I mean, these are normal things. But I don't do them.

Me: Exactly, I want this experience to feel like you are doing things that are normal but doubling down on the aspects of normal things that build up your circadian rhythms. I want you to do your normal day the way you do. And then I want you to add in getting outside or sitting near a window as much as you can during the day.

Alex: How about coffee? I need it to get through my classes.

Me: When do you usually finish drinking your coffee?

Alex: I have a cup of coffee after lunch to get through my afternoon classes. I'm usually done by three o'clock in the afternoon, I guess.

Me: Could you work that backward by a couple of hours? Caffeine stays in your system as long as ten full hours, with most of the effect happening in the first five hours.[66] The later in the day you drink it, the harder your circadian system has to work to compete with the caffeine to signal that it's time to rest.

Alex: What if I just finished the whole cup of coffee before 1:30 p.m.?

Me: That's better. Let's call it a bronze medal. Silver would be finishing before lunch. Gold would be coffee only before 9:00 a.m. And a double gold would be no coffee at all.

Alex: I'm never going to get a double gold; I'm telling you now.

Me: No worries. You are striving for some serious sleep medaling with your other efforts, and the bottom line is that you need to make this work for you and your lifestyle, not for me.

Alex: Okay, so I'm finishing caffeine before 1:30 p.m. Then what do I do?

## THE POWER IS OUT! IT'S TIME TO CAMP IN

One of the easiest ways to explain one of the core features of the Camping In Reset is to encourage people to think about it as coming home knowing the power has gone out in your home and it won't be back on until morning. There will be no lights, no television, no WiFi. You'll be using candles to see and maybe a flashlight if you need to do something technical.

Everyone understands what things are like when the power is out because we have all been there at one time or another. But the Camping In Reset has a few distinct advantages over the standard power outage. First, you know it's coming. That means you can prepare candles, better yet, battery-powered candles, twinkly lights, and one flashlight for your evening. Also, prepare your activities for the night. Craft projects are excellent, especially those that don't need bright light. But card games, board games, letter writing, grocery list making, laundry folding, even some yoga are all great activities.

Second, since the power isn't actually out, you still are able to use your heating and air conditioning, fans, and so on. Please do! Be comfortable. Also, you can charge your phone and not worry about whether the food will spoil in the fridge or when the power is coming back on like when the power is out.

There are many other layers to fully experience the Camping In Reset, but living evenings as if the power is out captures the essence of the work after sundown.

Me: It's your evenings that are going to be the most different. I want you to prepare for your evenings like you might **if you knew the power was going to go out at home.**

Alex: You want me to turn off the lights?

Me: More than that. When you get home at the end of the day, I want you not to turn on the lights. Keep the blinds and curtains open as wide as you like, get the candles and battery-powered lamps out, and prepare for a quiet night.

Alex: So, when it gets dark outside, it gets dark inside?

Me: Exactly. You are going to be living alongside the sun like most humans in history have.

Alex: Wait, why am I going to be living in the dark like most humans?

Me: Because your brain is built to follow the light and dark patterns, and they inform your circadian rhythms. All this effort will remind your brain that you are a normal human who follows the sun in the day and rests at night. For a million years, when it got dark, humans looked to rest. It's our modern experience that is different. You are going to spend two weeks reminding your brain that you aren't in a twenty-four-hour news cycle, or a twenty-four-hour TikTok cycle. You are active in the day and will be resting at night.

Alex: Okay, so living like a caveman.

Me: Or like Socrates, or Harriet Tubman, or Lincoln. Pick your favorite historical figure from before 1950, and you'll have this in common with them.

Alex: Okay, I get it. When it gets dark outside, it gets dark inside.

Me: Right. But before it gets dark outside, I'd like you to do the things you must get done with light. What would that be?

Alex: What do I do between getting home and going to bed? I eat dinner and text my mom. Most of my evenings I'm studying. But I also like to hang out with my roommates and my girlfriend. Sometimes we have *Mario Kart* tournaments together. And I like watching videos on YouTube. But I *have to* study. Can I do that with candlelight or a flashlight?

Me: I want you to prioritize your activities based on how essential light is. You can probably do *some* studying with low light, like a book light. But I think you'll find that it is tiring to study in low light. This means you'll need to be really focused on getting your studying done earlier, when the light is good. Remember, this is a two-week undertaking, not the rest of medical school.

Alex: Fair enough. Also, I just realized that I have two exams next week, so I may wait to start this.

Me: It's so important to think ahead like that. Make the timing of this work for you. Planning to start Camping In after your next two exams, when there is a little breathing room, is a great idea.

Alex: So, when I get started, I'll study and eat dinner as soon as I get home.

Me: Right. And what if instead of texting your mom during daylight, you just gave her a quick call to check in *after* sundown, so you use your evening light for studying? Would that work?

Alex: I could do that for a couple of weeks, sure. My mom will thank you.

Me: And then we need to consider how you'll spend your evenings with your roommates and your girlfriend. They may not all want to spend their evenings in the dark on your timetable.

Alex: Yeah, I don't think any of them will want to do that.

Me: I've been surprised how many partners and roommates have gotten interested in this idea and joined in, but you know your roommates and I don't. How about your girlfriend? Will she be able to support this?

Alex: Yeah, totally. Also, one of my roommates will be totally into this; she loves sleep hacks. But the other one is glued to her phone and TikTok, so I'm thinking she's not going to be on board. My girlfriend stays with me on the weekends, and I think she would be good with this—she really wants me to sleep better.

Me: Those are the three people I want you to talk to before you start, so they are all on the same page with you. And if the whole apartment doesn't want to join you in this, that's okay; you just need to find space where you can have the dark.

Alex: Okay, I'll talk to them. I only have my phone for a flashlight, and I'm getting the sense that's not really what you have in mind.

Me: I'd love for you to have some battery-powered lamps with soft light to spend your evenings with. Some people call them *twinkly lights*. My favorites are the kind that look like they are candles but are battery powered. You can find inexpensive ones online. If you can have two or three, or even four of them, then there is more gentle light. It still is unlikely to be enough light to study in for long.

Alex: You haven't said what time I'm supposed to go to bed yet. Isn't that a big part of this?

Me: You usually go to bed at midnight, right?

Alex: Yeah, though I wish I could fall asleep earlier than that.

Me: Here's the thing. We are training your circadian rhythms with this plan. When they are strong, they will let you know when it's time to go to bed. I want you to go to bed when you are sleepy and let your body guide you.

Alex: That's it? You aren't giving me a bedtime?

Me: After a few nights of having evenings in the relative dark, your brain will be clear about bedtime coming soon.

This will become something you don't need to think about much.

Alex: That would be amazing, but I'll believe it when I see it. Also, how will I know when I'm sleepy and not just tired?

Me: You know that feeling when your eyes feel heavy or droopy and you aren't thinking so clearly, like you are about to nod off?

Alex: Oh, yeah. That's something I know well.

Me: That's sleepiness, pure and simple. You may notice other things like frequent yawning, forgetting what you were reading, and difficulty getting yourself to do anything. These are all signs it's sleepiness, not just feeling tired.

Alex: Okay, I know those things. And then I'll get myself to bed.

Me: It can take a good number of days before you get there, but it will happen. On the flip side, the time you wake up each day is vital. A consistent wake time is a strong signal to your brain and body that it's time to get started. The more closely you stick to your wake time, the better all of this will go.

Alex: I remember. And that makes sense to me now.

Me: What we didn't talk much about is how you are going to spend your evenings when you aren't watching YouTube or doing *Mario Kart* tournaments.

Alex: Oh, right. If I get done studying early and then it's dark and the "power is out," I'm not playing video games or using my laptop, am I?

Me: Right. You are going to be spending your evenings doing things more like your grandparents probably did.

Alex: Can I talk on the phone as long as I'm not playing on my phone?

Me: Did your grandparents talk on the phone after sundown?

Alex: Yep. I see what you are saying.

Me: What else can you think of to do?

Alex: They played cards together, and I like playing cards. Actually, I really like crocheting, but I haven't done it for a while. My girlfriend and I like playing Scrabble.

Me: These are all excellent ideas. They all work great. This may sound old, but you could write letters and notes to people in your life. You could get a bunch of postcards and write one or two each night to friends. Or you could write a letter and mail it to someone you haven't seen in a while.

Alex: What a strange idea. Lol. My old college roommate would love to get a letter from me. Also, my roommate has a record player. That seems like something I could do without using lights. Is that fine to do?

Me: Absolutely, listening to music is a great wind down activity. And a record player means you don't have to look at a screen to use it. How likely do you feel you can follow through with this plan?

Alex: There isn't anything hard about this, other than getting my studying mostly done before dark. But I need to know my girlfriend is going to be on board with it, and I need to see how my roommates are going to react. If they aren't on board, it's going to be harder.

## PREPARE YOUR SOCIAL NETWORK

It's very important to the Camping In Reset to have the people in your social world aware of what you are doing, especially those with whom you share space during the evenings: roommates, significant others and partners. When you let them know, be clear that you aren't looking for their approval, but that it will be very helpful if they were able to work with you for two weeks by not being disruptive to your process.

You are changing the lighting and the electronic and digital activities for yourself for these two weeks. Having your family or roommates join in is the best-case scenario, but it's not always going to happen. Be prepared for that possibility. You may need to spend more time apart from people whom you care about but who aren't willing or aren't able to join you in Camping In. Remind yourself of your motivations for trying and the struggles that have led you to this point. If you are pleasantly surprised that you will have company in Camping In, all the better. But if you are prepared to Camp In by yourself or with little support, you will be ready for just about anything.

Me: I'm going to guess that your roommates are going to be partially on board, and that's better than not at all. I want you to talk with them and then figure out how to make it work alongside their lives.

Alex: That's my next step, then. Talking to all of them about what I want to do. And you are promising me that I'll be sleeping well within two weeks of starting this, right?

Me: There are no promises because everyone is different. However, most people who undertake this with my guidance have found that within a few days they are feeling calmer, and within a week, their sleep feels more natural, like a rhythm, and less like something they are chasing.

Alex: Okay, can I check in with you in about a week when I've talked to my roommates? I'm not planning to start this until after my exams next Tuesday.

Me: Let's talk Wednesday.

Alex: Perfect, that will help me get it all settled before starting.

Me: Let me give you these nine basic guidelines to take with you when you talk to your girlfriend and roommates.

## CAMPING-IN RESET GUIDELINES:

1. Wake up at the same time every day and get out of bed within a few minutes.
2. Keep your window blinds mostly open.
3. Eat and drink something about an hour after you wake up.
4. Go about your day and be outside or near windows as much as possible.
5. In the evening, keep the lights in your house turned off before sundown.
6. As sundown approaches, use small battery-powered lamps for light, but mostly let the darkness be darkness.
7. After sundown, operate as if there were a power outage—no TV, no internet use, and no phone use other than actual phone calls. Use an actual flashlight (not your phone) for activities that demand vision (like the bathroom).
8. Before bedtime, stay out of bed and enjoy activities like your grandparents might have: playing card games (like solitaire and gin rummy), doing crosswords, reading with a booklight, working on craft projects under lower light (crocheting, knitting, coloring, etc.), folding laundry, trying those exercises your physical therapist wants you to do, calling a friend, playing Bananagrams or Scrabble, writing a letter to an old friend, or anything else that fits with these activities.
9. When you feel sleepy, not just tired, it's time for bed. Make sure the blinds or curtains to your bedroom window are at least partially open to allow sunlight to come

into the room in the morning. If there is overnight light from outside (for instance, if your window is near a streetlight), keep your blinds or curtains closed at night, but open them immediately upon waking.

## WEDNESDAY

Alex: Hi, Doc. I've got some questions for you!

Me: Welcome back, Alex. How were your exams?

Alex: Not bad; I'm glad they are done. I'm tired from all that studying, but I don't have another exam for a few weeks.

Me: Glad to hear it. How are you feeling about getting the camp-in started?

Alex: I'm a little nervous, but I think I'm all set to start tonight.

Me: Excellent! How did the conversations with your girlfriend and roommates go?

Alex: I was surprised how on board with the plans my girlfriend is. She has all kinds of ideas for playing games and calling friends together after I finish studying. My roommates were just like I thought they would be. Allison wants to do the whole thing herself, too, and Janessa wants nothing to do with it.

Me: You completely expected that, which is hilarious.

Alex: Well, we've known each other for a long time.

Me: So how will you, Allison, and your girlfriend work with Janessa?

Alex: Well, Janessa works late two nights a week, and by the time she gets home, I'm just about ready for bed. So, on those nights, I'll just head to my bedroom before she gets home. On the other nights, she's agreed to do the power-out routine for an hour with me, but then she wants to watch her shows. At that point, I'll go to my room or sit outside if it's nice enough out.

Me: That sounds reasonable. I'm glad you found a way to work together on this.

Alex: If I were doing this for more than two weeks, I think Janessa might have blown a fuse. The fact that it's just a couple of weeks and she is leaving town for one of those weekends made this pretty easy. But I was surprised that Allison wants to try this as her new reset, too. She's in med school with me and loves the idea.

Me: You mentioned you were a little nervous about starting. Anything I can help with?

Alex: Mostly, I'm nervous about studying enough before it gets dark. I know I can study with a book light and I'm planning to do that, but I imagine I'll only be able to do that for an hour or so.

Me: I think you're right about studying for an hour with the booklight. You may get more time than that, but the booklight's tiring for your mind and your eyes. I have confidence in you staying focused on getting most of the work done before dark. Did you ever have a job during high school or college?

Alex: Yeah, I worked at a restaurant one year during high school.

Me: Did anyone tell you that having that job would make it harder to get all your schoolwork done?

Alex: Oh yeah, they really did. I needed to spend twenty hours a week doing this job to make some money, but I also thought I was going to struggle to keep up with school.

Me: And what happened?

Alex: It was fine. I had to be more focused on getting my work done, but I was fine. So you're saying studying before dark can be like that?

Me: The work of medical school is more demanding than high school work, but yes, that's what I'm saying. You are going to be really focused on getting that work done. Sleep helps you store and retain memory, and the restfulness you get from the resetting of your circadian rhythms will help your brain as well once you get back on track. Also, I think it was wise to wait until after your exams ended to start this. What other concerns do you have?

Alex: I'm a little concerned about falling asleep. I can't imagine that I'll be tired enough to fall asleep after just playing cards and talking with my friends, but I guess that's what I used to do when I was a kid, and I slept better back then.

Me: I know you have been taking an hour or so to fall asleep, but the new plan should help you feel relaxed and calmer before bed and you won't be getting into bed until you are feeling sleepy, not just tired. It may take a couple of nights to get into your flow, your routine, but I'm hoping it won't feel like effort. And you already wake up too early, so waking up and starting your day at the same time shouldn't be challenging.

Alex: That's true. And, well, it all starts tonight.

Me: I'd love to check in with you in a week, when you are halfway through. How does that sound?

Alex: Great. I can't wait to find out what happens.

### Two Weeks Later

And Alex was on her way. She had to cancel her appointment the following week when something came up, but we met after her thirteenth night, and she had a big smile on her face.

She explained that it had been a challenge, but that it had been worth it. The biggest challenge was what she worried it would be: falling asleep at the start of the night. For the first few nights, she still needed over an hour to fall asleep. But there were surprising wins that she wanted to tell me about.

> Alex: I thought this was such a crazy idea, and I have to admit, my expectations were low. "Just turn off the lights and you'll sleep better" sounded way too good to be true.
>
> Me: I couldn't agree more—it sounds too easy. But what happened?
>
> Alex: Well, first, I learned to study right after class. I decided to stay on campus and study there because I can get home later without burning daylight. I just packed an extra snack, said goodbye to my classmates at the end of the day, and settled into studying. It worked well because there were no distractions. I had to stay focused, but after a few days, it was my new routine, and it wasn't bad. I would usually stay for three or four hours, which is basically all the time I was studying before this anyway.
>
> Me: Excellent. You found a great strategy to make it work for you.
>
> Alex: Doing that meant the pressure to study in low light was gone. I always left campus before sundown, and I was home in time to get the battery lamps out. We found some of those battery-operated candle lamps—they are nice.

Me: And how were your evenings?

Alex: I can't believe how relaxed I felt. I felt like there was nothing to do for the first time in months. And it was easy to catch up on little household chores like laundry, dishes, and putting things away. The apartment was cleaner than ever. But I was so relaxed.

Me: That's the main thing I hear from people who try this—how relaxing it is to "camp in" or have the "power out." You were concerned before you started about falling asleep being difficult. How did that go?

Alex: Yeah, it wasn't great for the first three nights. I was relaxed getting into bed, so I didn't feel stress like I do sometimes, but I used some of the breathing techniques you told me about and the counting thing—Counting for Sleep—and eventually I got to sleep. But by the weekend, so about the fourth night, I fell asleep in thirty minutes instead of an hour. Over the second week it took me less and less time to fall asleep. Like last night I think it took me about fifteen minutes.

Me: That's great progress. The national average for time to fall asleep is fifteen minutes for healthy adults, so welcome to the land of normal sleep onset times.

Alex: I had no idea that Camping In would work that well for this. Falling asleep was always my biggest problem when I was dealing with insomnia. Oh, I nearly forgot to mention that this second week I've been going to bed earlier, usually like 11:00 p.m., and still falling asleep within fifteen minutes. I did what you said and listened to my body. I went to bed when I felt sleepy—like my eyes were drooping so I went to bed.

Me: Amazing. That's another thing that tends to happen to a lot of people who do the Camping In—they feel relaxed, they feel a little bored, and their body starts to encourage them to get to bed.

Alex: That's just how it felt.

Me: Two other things—how was waking up, and how was your fatigue throughout the days?

Alex: Right. The first few days, while I was still struggling to fall asleep, it was challenging to finish my coffee at 1:30 p.m. and then last the rest of the afternoon without any caffeine while still feeling tired. I kept reminding myself that it's just for two weeks, and that I didn't have any exams on the near horizon. If I got drowsy, I'd get up from studying and walk around for a bit. Sometimes I did jumping jacks.

Me: I'm glad you could pull that off. I know it's no small task, especially when you are trying to keep up with medical school.

Alex: I also started taking a snack with me and would eat that about an hour after I woke up, and I took my lunch outside every day. Well, one day it was raining hard, so I ate in front of the big front windows of our building. But every other day someone went outside for lunch with me. That was different from my typical lunch of scrolling and texting while I sat in a room with one window.

Me: You were boosting your circadian rhythms with all the blue light from the sun. That's great! Did it feel any different to you?

Alex: Not at first—it felt like a chore. But after a few days, I looked forward to it. And my friends started to join me, and now I eat outside most of the time.

Me: Fantastic. This is so good for you and for your friends!

Alex: Some of them are scrolling their phones while they eat, but at least we are outside, right?

Me: Absolutely. Any other added outside time in your days?

Alex: Yep. In the afternoon, before my last class of the day, I would take a ten-minute walk outside. I'd call someone to chat or just walk and let my mind wander.

Me: This is gold medal Camping In you are telling me about. I'm really proud of how well you did this.

Alex: If it took the full two weeks to feel improvement, I'm not sure I would have made it. But I started falling asleep more easily after a few nights, and my morning sleep lasted almost until my alarm after about five or six days. So, overall, I was getting a bit more sleep than I had been before this started, which meant I was less tired in the afternoons.

Me: It sounds like it was beginning to work well for you after about five or six days.

Alex: That's right. And we learned that my roommate Janessa likes playing hearts, so we convinced her to sit with the battery lamps and play hearts a couple of nights rather than watch TV. It was fun, and being separate on the other nights was fine. Also, I wrote a letter to my old roommate. It was nice!

Me: See—your grandparents didn't have it so bad, did they?

Alex: I'm not throwing away my phone or anything, but it wasn't as hard as I expected. Some nights I got a little bored, but I started to appreciate feeling bored. With studying, looking at my phone, and watching all the shows people recommend, I haven't felt bored in a long time. Now I realize that I've been feeling a little overwhelmed by all the stuff. So the break was refreshing. We had fun most of the time, and like I said, it was relaxing.

Alex told me that her roommates were in and out of the Camping In action—sometimes they were hanging out and playing cards and chatting; other nights they wanted to watch TV or play video games, and those nights were harder because it would have been so easy just to join them and hang out. Alex instead reminded herself that it was "just for two weeks" and went to her room to call her mom or girlfriend or write a postcard.

She also explained that her girlfriend and her roommate Allison did the Camping In alongside her on more than one night. They were curious about it and had a *why not?* attitude. That made it a lot more fun.

In the end, this was the intervention Alex needed. It helped her reset and power up her circadian rhythms so that sleep became more routine, easier to anticipate, and easier to enjoy. An unexpected positive effect for Alex was that it helped her condense her study time in a focused period. This had the double benefit of allowing her to take the rest of her evenings off from studying as well as encouraging relaxation, both things that promote better sleep.

Alex, like most people I've worked with who tried it, found Camping In to be easier than she expected. She also expressed an interest in doing it again. Alex thought she might do it one week out of every month. Others who have appreciated its effects have begun to use it once a week or every Monday and Tuesday.

There really is no downside to Camping In. I've never met anyone who wanted to change their lives and "camp in" every night, but I imagine they are out there somewhere. If that's you, send me a message—I'd love to hear about your process and maybe help you with any questions. Or maybe you can help me learn more from your extensive experience.

One of the most frequent pushbacks I get from people who are considering it is how they will keep up with the news or social media posts from their friends. My response? Give it a try for one night. That night, estimate how much time you would have needed to spend if you hadn't "camped in" without social media before you go to bed. Then, when you wake up, time yourself for how long it takes to actually catch up on those posts. I think you'll be surprised that it's much less time than if you had kept up during the night. One client of mine found that the hour of social media she consumed before bed translated into about ninety seconds of catching up the next morning. Your mileage may vary, but I expect you'll find it to be a net gain on your time and effort.

### The Refrigerator Interrogation

The biggest surprise for me and most others who "camp in" has been the shocking brightness of the light in your refrigerator. When the lights are turned off and your eyes aren't ready for it, opening the fridge can feel like an interrogation light. Luckily, your fridge probably has a workaround for this.

If you observe the Sabbath on Friday nights, you know all about this. Ryann, a colleague of mine, heard about my interrogation fridge lights while I was talking about Camping In and told me to use the *Sabbath mode* on my fridge. She explained that my fridge has a built-in mode I never knew about, but millions of Jewish people do. She told me how to use it. I love learning something new.

Orthodox Jews do not use electricity, including lights in the fridge, during their weekly observance of the Sabbath. But they aren't going to let all the food in the fridge spoil. Modern refrigerators generally have a built-in code to turn the fridge light off for seventy-two to eighty-five hours while the fridge otherwise remains fully functional. You can also turn Sabbath mode off when you are done using it. In my household, that's the morning after you are done Camping In.

Search the internet for "Sabbath Mode" instructions for your refrigerator and if you have an older model without a code, prepare yourself before opening that fridge door.

### Is Camping In for Me?

Alex and Lee had distinct sleep problems. Each was a little bit desperate to find a pathway to better sleep. Each had a history of insomnia, but their current sleep problems didn't meet the criteria for an insomnia diagnosis. Lee's Camping Out Sleep Reset and Alex's Camping In worked for them. What about you?

Since developing this idea, I've recommended it to dozens of people. Although all of them describe feeling tired during the day, every day, these are otherwise people who have no sleep disorders or sleep problems other than the normal "bad night of sleep from time to time." So, they are probably a bit like you. Their response to Camping In has been positive. The most common response I get from people is that it helps them feel more relaxed and they often go to sleep earlier than usual.

Here are my recommendations for how you can try this out at home:

1. **Talk** with your partner, roommate, older children, and any other members of your household whose lives will be affected. They don't need to join you 100%, but they need to be on board with your process. If they join you, even for part of the time, all the better!
2. **Commit** to Camping In for more than one night. Two nights is a great start, and three is even better. After you "camp in" once or twice you can switch to a single Camping In night periodically, maybe even weekly. But the first time you do it I strongly recommend at least two nights so that your body gets a more complete experience and the impact is stronger.
3. **Prepare** for your nights. Make sure you have batteries in the flashlight, but more importantly, get yourself some low-light lamps. Some people call them "twinkle lights," other people call them "fairy lights," but if you do an internet search for either term, you'll see what I'm talking about. These are very gentle lights that provide enough light to see the cards you are playing hearts with but not bright at all. These will be your go-to lights. I like them to be battery powered so I can walk around with them. I discourage actual candles because fire isn't the safest thing—and no one ever

caught their hair on fire with battery-powered twinkle lights or battery-powered candles.

4. **Plan** for your mornings. Know what time you will be out of bed no matter how you slept. The sun streaming in your window should be helpful. If you wait to figure this out as you are waking up, you will be tempted to stay in bed longer, and you don't want that because the morning start is a strong component to kick-starting your circadian rhythms.
5. **Anticipate** your daytime activities. Camping In means daytime too! Plan for how you will get your extra sunshine during the day—the more the better because it strengthens your circadian rhythms, making it easier to get sleepy at night. Plan ahead for when you will end your caffeine use during the day. Prepare for how you will adjust your schedule to allow for better afternoons. Maybe you need to take a five-minute outdoor walk before your late afternoon meetings or classes.
6. **Get excited!** This is your chance to do those things you never really make time to do when you are busy with catching up on shows, watching YouTube and TikTok videos, and generally just staying busy. For me, it's crossword puzzles from the local newspaper. For Alex it was playing hearts with her roommates. Lee was alone most of the time, and he read books and wrote letters. What will it be for you? Don't just plan to do chores (a few are fine) but be sure to have something to look forward to. These nights can feel a little daunting without some fun planned.

# CONCLUSION

We arrived here by recognizing a simple truth: Modern life pulls against how human bodies were built to sleep. In evolutionary terms, the leap from campfire nights to twenty-four-hour lights, cable TV, and endlessly engaging screens happened in the blink of an eye, and our rhythms haven't caught up. Along the way, a well-funded *Sleep Better Now!* marketplace promised quick fixes, selling us pillows, potions, and dashboards for a biological drive we already possess. This book has asked you to look past that noise and return to first principles: protecting your rhythms and letting sleep do what sleep is designed to do.

The foundation is this: Sleep is a drive, like hunger, thirst, and breathing. Because it is a drive, it is resilient; your body will seek it and take it given the chance. Our big, brilliant human brains complicate things by worrying about sleep and worry itself is one of the fastest ways to trip the very system we're trying to support. The work, then, is not to force sleep but to get out of its way.

As a practical reset, we explored Camping Out (when you can) and Camping In (any time), not just for fun but as structured ways to re-expose your brain to the signals it expects: bright days, dim and quiet evenings, and fewer late-night decisions. Even small at-home moves—gentler light, a steadier morning, fewer nighttime interruptions (down to the refrigerator light)—restore rhythm.

And we kept returning to the mindset. Insomnia expands when fear fills the gaps; it recedes when you replace catastrophic stories with tested facts and patient practice. The goal isn't to assemble a flawless "cookie recipe" for perfect nights—it's to become a steadier surfer, catching the next wave when the last one passes you by.

If you're a clinician, coach, educator, or leader, you now have a language and levers that translate across settings, from campus to clinic to locker room to boardroom. If you're simply tired of being tired, you have enough to begin today without buying anything—just aligning what you do with what your body already knows.

I wrote this because sleep changed my life, first through a medical fix that let me breathe and then through years of watching healthy rhythms lift people out of fog and back into themselves. That's why the message is hopeful: Your biology and your body want to help you. Give them light in the morning, quiet at night, and a little grace in between. Remember: "Your body will get the sleep it needs, even if you get in the way."

# GREAT BOOKS ABOUT SLEEP AND CIRCADIAN RHYTHMS

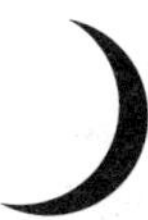

Aschwanden, Christie. *Good to Go: What the Athlete in All of Us Can Learn from the Strange Science of Recovery*. New York: W. W. Norton & Company, 2019.

Ehrnstrom, Colleen, and Alisha L. Brosse. *End the Insomnia Struggle: A Step-by-Step Guide to Help You Get to Sleep and Stay Asleep.* Oakland, CA: New Harbinger Publications, 2016.

Hersey, Tricia. *Rest Is Resistance: A Manifesto.* New York: Little, Brown Spark, 2022.

Leibowitz, Kari. *How to Winter.* New York: Portfolio, 2024.

Lembke, Anna. *Dopamine Nation: Finding Balance in the Age of Indulgence.* New York: Dutton, 2021.

Macedo, Diane. *The Sleep Fix: Practical, Proven, and Surprising Solutions for Insomnia, Snoring, Shift Work, and More*. New York: HarperCollins, 2021.

Mendelson, Wallace B. *The Science of Sleep: What It Is, How It Works, and Why It Matters*. Chicago: University of Chicago Press, 2017.

Nestor, James. *Breath: The New Science of a Lost Art*. New York: Riverhead Books, 2020.

Pollan, Michael. *Caffeine: How Caffeine Created the Modern World*. New York: Audible Originals, 2019.

Price, Catherine. *How to Break Up with Your Phone: The 30-Day Plan to Take Back Your Life*. New York: Ten Speed Press, 2025.

Rosen, Larry D., and Adam Gazzaley. *The Distracted Mind: Ancient Brains in a High-Tech World*. Cambridge, MA: MIT Press, 2016.

Stuart-Smith, Sue. *The Well-Gardened Mind: The Restorative Power of Nature*. New York: Scribner, 2020.

Twenge, Jean M. *iGen: Why Today's Super-Connected Kids Are Growing Up Less Rebellious, More Tolerant, Less Happy—and Completely Unprepared for Adulthood—and What That Means for the Rest of Us*. New York: Atria Books, 2018.

Winter, W. Chris. *The Sleep Solution: Why Your Sleep Is Broken and How to Fix It*. New York: Berkley, 2017.

# NOTES

1 Benjafield, A. V., Ayas, N. T., Eastwood, P. R., Heinzer, R., Ip, M. S. M., Morrell, M. J., Nunez, C. M., Patel, S. R., Penzel, T., Pépin, J. L., Peppard, P. E., Sinha, S., Tufik, S., Valentine, K., & Malhotra, A. (2019). Estimation of the global prevalence and burden of obstructive sleep apnoea: a literature-based analysis. *The Lancet*. Respiratory medicine, 7(8), 687–698. https://doi.org/10.1016/S2213-2600(19)30198-5

2 Hibberd, T. J., Ramsay, S., Spencer-Merris, P., Dinning, P. G., Zagorodnyuk, V. P., & Spencer, N. J. (2023). Circadian rhythms in colonic function. *Frontiers in physiology*, 14, 1239278. https://doi.org/10.3389/fphys.2023.1239278

3 Samson, D. R., Crittenden, A. N., Mabulla, I. A., Mabulla, A. Z. P., & Nunn, C. L. (2017). Chronotype variation drives night-time sentinel-like behaviour in hunter-gatherers. Proceedings. *Biological sciences*, 284(1858), 20170967. https://doi.org/10.1098/rspb.2017.0967

4 Hagenauer, M. H., Perryman, J. I., Lee, T. M., & Carskadon, M. A. (2009). Adolescent changes in the homeostatic and circadian regulation of sleep. *Developmental neuroscience*, 31(4), 276–284. https://doi.org/10.1159/000216538

5 Boyce N. (2023). Have we lost sleep? A reconsideration of segmented sleep in early modern England. *Medical history*, 67(2), 91–108. https://doi.org/10.1017/mdh.2023.14

6 Cottle, S. (2017, May 20). An early history of lighting in NYC. Milrose Consultants. Retrieved August 31, 2025, from https://www.milrose.com/insights/an-early-history-of-lighting-in-nyc

7 Ojomo, E. (2024, August 22). How the history of electrification in the United States can help The World Bank's ambitious plan to electrify Africa. Clayton Christensen Institute. Retrieved August 31, 2025, from https://www.christenseninstitute.org/blog/how-the-history-of-electrification-in-the-united-states-can-help-the-world-banks-ambitious-plan-to-electrify-africa/

8 Martin, S. (1977). Closing. On *Let's get small* [Comedy album]. Warner Bros. Records.

9 Montgomery, A. (2024, January 28). Lessons from sleeplessness: The 60th anniversary of Randy Gardner's world record. NPR. Retrieved August 31, 2025, from https://www.npr.org/2024/01/28/1227217274/sleep-deprivation-record#:~:text=The%20news%20made%20its%20way,actually%20won%20all%20the%20time

10 Matthews, C. E., Chen, K. Y., Freedson, P. S., Buchowski, M. S., Beech, B., Pate, R. R., & Troiano, R. P. (2008). Amount of time spent in sedentary behaviors in the United States, 2003–2004. *American Journal of Epidemiology*, 167(7), 875–881. https://doi.org/10.1093/aje/kwm390

11 U.S. Environmental Protection Agency. (2025, April 9). Improving your indoor environment. Retrieved January 13, 2026, from https://www.epa.gov/indoor-air-quality-iaq/improving-your-indoor-environment

12 Occupational Safety and Health Administration. (n.d.). Indoor air quality in commercial and institutional buildings (Publication No. 3430). U.S. Department of Labor. Retrieved January 13, 2026, from https://www.osha.gov/sites/default/files/publications/3430indoor-air-quality-sm.pdf

13 Mindell, J. A., Bartle, A., Abd Wahab, N., Ahn, Y., Ramamurthy, M. B., Huong, H. T. D., Kohyama, J., Ruangdaraganon, N., Sekartini, R., Teng, A., & Goh, D. Y. (2011). Sleep education in medical school curriculum: a glimpse across countries. *Sleep medicine*, 12(9), 928-931.

14 Substance Abuse and Mental Health Services Administration, Center for Behavioral Health Statistics and Quality. (2013, May 1). Emergency department visits for adverse reactions involving the insomnia medication zolpidem (The DAWN Report). U.S. Department of Health and Human Services.

15 U.S. Food and Drug Administration. (2019, April 30). FDA adds Boxed Warning for risk of serious injuries caused by sleepwalking with certain prescription insomnia medicines. https://www.fda.gov/drugs/drug-safety-and-availability/fda-adds-boxed-warning-risk-seri-

ous-injuries-caused-sleepwalking-certain-prescription-insomnia

16 Pawar, R. S., Coppin, J. P., Khanna, S., & Parker, C. H. (2025). A Survey of Melatonin in Dietary Supplement Products Sold in the United States. *Drug testing and analysis*, 17(8), 1176–1185. https://doi.org/10.1002/dta.3823

17 Dement, W., & Kleitman, N. (1957). Cyclic variations in EEG during sleep and their relation to eye movements, body motility, and dreaming. *Electroencephalography and Clinical Neurophysiology*, 9(4), 673–690. https://doi.org/10.1016/0013-4694(57)90088-3

18 Axelsson, J., Sundelin, T., Ingre, M., Van Someren, E. J. W., Olsson, A., & Lekander, M. (2010). Beauty sleep: Experimental study on the perceived health and attractiveness of sleep-deprived people. *BMJ*, 341, c6614. https://doi.org/10.1136/bmj.c6614

19 Sundelin, T., Lekander, M., Sorjonen, K., & Axelsson, J. (2017). Negative effects of restricted sleep on facial appearance and social appeal. Royal Society Open Science, 4(5), 160918. https://doi.org/10.1098/rsos.160918

20 Gresser, D., McLimans, K., Lee, S., & Morgan-Bathke, M. (2025). The Impact of Sleep Deprivation on Hunger-Related Hormones: A Meta-Analysis and Systematic Review. *Obesities*, 5(2), 48. https://doi.org/10.3390/obesities5020048

21 Sleep Foundation. (2025, July 11). How much sleep do you really need? Sleep Foundation. Retrieved September 7, 2025, from https://www.sleepfoundation.org/how-sleep-works/how-much-sleep-do-we-really-need

22 Short, M. A., Gradisar, M., Wright, H., Lack, L. C., Dohnt, H., & Carskadon, M. A. (2011). Time for bed: parent-set bedtimes associated with improved sleep and daytime functioning in adolescents. *Sleep*, 34(6), 797–800. https://doi.org/10.5665/SLEEP.1052

23 Sleep Foundation. (n.d.). How much sleep do you really need? Retrieved January 13, 2026, from https://www.sleepfoundation.org/how-sleep-works/how-much-sleep-do-we-really-need

24 Kripke, D. F., Garfinkel, L., Wingard, D. L., Klauber, M. R., & Marler, M. R. (2002). Mortality associated with sleep duration and insomnia. *Archives of General Psychiatry*, 59(2), 131–136. https://doi.org/10.1001/archpsyc.59.2.131

25 Berg, S. (2022, April 1). What doctors wish patients knew about sleep apnea. American Medical Association. Retrieved September 7, 2025, from https://www.ama-assn.org/delivering-care/prevention-wellness/what-doctors-wish-patients-knew-about-sleep-apnea

26 Ghavami, T., Kazeminia, M., Ahmadi, N., & Rajati, F. (2023). Global Prevalence of Obstructive Sleep Apnea in the Elderly and Related Factors: A Systematic Review and Meta-Analysis Study. *Journal of perianesthesia nursing*: official journal of the American Society of

PeriAnesthesia Nurses, 38(6), 865–875. https://doi.org/10.1016/j.jopan.2023.01.018

27 Dancey, D. R., Hanly, P. J., Soong, C., Lee, B., & Hoffstein, V. (2001). Impact of menopause on the prevalence and severity of sleep apnea. *Chest*, 120(1), 151–155. https://doi.org/10.1378/chest.120.1.151

28 There are many other studies that have shown the same results. These three citations just scratch the surface:

Jullian-Desayès, I., et al. (2016). Impact of concomitant medications on obstructive sleep apnoea: opioids cause relaxation of the tongue and upper airway muscles... *British Journal of Clinical Pharmacology*.

Hsu, T.-W., Chen, H.-M., Chen, T.-Y., Chu, C.-S., & Pan, C.-C. (2021). The association between use of benzodiazepine receptor agonists and the risk of obstructive sleep apnea: A nationwide population-based nested case–control study. *International Journal of Environmental Research and Public Health*, 18(18), 9720.

Wang, S. H., et al. (2019). Benzodiazepines associated with acute respiratory failure in OSA patients. *Frontiers in Pharmacology*.

29 Ambesh, P., Shetty, V., Ambesh, S., Gupta, S. S., Kamholz, S., & Wolf, L. (2018). Jet lag: Heuristics and therapeutics. *Journal of family medicine and primary care*, 7(3), 507–510. https://doi.org/10.4103/jfmpc.jfmpc_220_17

30 Hussey KD. Timeless spaces: Field experiments in the physiological study of circadian rhythms, 1938-1963. *Hist Philos Life Sci.* 2023 Apr 19;45(2):17. doi: 10.1007/s40656-023-00571-w. PMID: 37076757; PMCID: PMC10115684.

31 Mills, J. N. (1964). Circadian rhythms during and after three months in solitude underground. *The Journal of Physiology*, 174(2), 217–231.

Halberg F., Siffre M., Engeli M., Hillman D., Reinberg A. Etude en libre-cours des rythmes circadiens du pouls, de l'alternance veille-sommeil et de l'estimation du temps pendant les deux mois de s'ejour souterrain d'un homme adulte jeune [free-run study of circadian rhythms of the pulse, of waking-sleep alternation and estimation of time during the 2 months of subterranean sojourn of a young adult male]. *C R Hebd Seances Acad Sci.* 1965 Jan 25;260:1259-62. Italian. PMID: 14275971.

32 Blume C, Garbazza C, Spitschan M. Effects of light on human circadian rhythms, sleep and mood. *Somnologie* (Berl). 2019 Sep;23(3):147-156. doi: 10.1007/s11818-019-00215-x. Epub 2019 Aug 20. PMID: 31534436; PMCID: PMC6751071.

33 Downs, S. (2022, June 29). *A Survey of Modern Life: Outdoor Time*. Building H. Retrieved from Medium.

34 U.S. Census Bureau. (1975). *Historical Statistics of the United States, Colonial Times to 1970, Part 1*. Washington, DC: U.S. Government Printing Office.

35 Miller, G. A. (1956). The magical number seven, plus or minus two: Some limits on our capacity for processing information. *Psychological Review*, 63(2), 81–97.

36 Cowan, N. (2001). The magical number 4 in short-term memory: A reconsideration of mental storage capacity. *Behavioral and Brain Sciences*, 24(1), 87–185.

37 Burke, T. M., Markwald, R. R., McHill, A. W., Chinoy, E. D., Snider, J. B., Bessman, S. C., ... & Czeisler, C. A. (2015). Effects of caffeine on the human circadian clock in vivo and in vitro. *Science Translational Medicine*, 7(305), 305ra146. https://doi.org/10.1126/scitranslmed.aac5125

38 Ruby, C. L., Brager, A. J., DePaul, M. A., Prosser, R. A., & Glass, J. D. (2018). Chronic caffeine consumption disrupts the circadian timing system. *Chronobiology International*, 35(12), 1614–1628. https://doi.org/10.1080/07420528.2018.1498928

39 Rosekind, M. R., Graeber, R. C., Dinges, D. F., Connell, L. J., & Rountree, M. S. (1994). Crew factors in flight operations IX: Effects of planned cockpit rest on crew performance and alertness in long-haul operations. NASA Ames Research Center.

40 Harvard Health Publishing. (2022, September 1). Can a quick snooze help with energy and focus? The science behind power naps. Harvard Medical School.

41 Hughes, N., & Burke, J. (2018). Sleeping with the frenemy: How restricting 'bedroom use' of smartphones impacts happiness and wellbeing. *Computers in Human Behavior*, 85, 236–244. https://doi.org/10.1016/j.chb.2018.03.047

42 Islam, M., Ahmed, O., & Islam, M. (2025). Linking nighttime smartphone location, sleep quality, and depressive symptoms in Bangladeshi young adults: The mediating role of bedtime smartphone use. *Journal of Technology in Behavioral Science*. Advance online publication. https://doi.org/10.1007/s41347-025-00536-9

43 Koh, G. K., Ow Yong, J. Q. Y., Lee, A. R. Y. B., Ong, B. S. Y., Yau, C. E., Ho, C. S. H., & Goh, Y. S. (2024). Social media use and its impact on adults' mental health and well-being: A scoping review. *Worldviews on evidence-based nursing*, 21(4), 345–394. https://doi.org/10.1111/wvn.12727

44 Lopes, L. S., Valentini, J. P., Monteiro, T. H., Costacurta, M. C. F., Soares, L. O. N., Telfar-Barnard, L., & Nunes, P. V. (2022). Problem-

atic Social Media Use and Its Relationship with Depression or Anxiety: A Systematic Review. *Cyberpsychology, behavior and social networking*, 25(11), 691–702. https://doi.org/10.1089/cyber.2021.0300

45 Jahagirdar, V., Sequeira, L. A., Kinattingal, N., & et al. (2024). Assessment of the impact of social media addiction on psychosocial behaviour like depression, stress, and anxiety in working professionals. *BMC Psychology*, 12, 352. https://doi.org/10.1186/s40359-024-01850-2

46 Nesi, J., Burke, T. A., Bettis, A. H., Kudinova, A. Y., Thompson, E. C., MacPherson, H. A., Fox, K. A., Aguilera, A., & Liu, R. T. (2021). Social media use and self-injurious thoughts and behaviors: A systematic review and meta-analysis. *Clinical Psychology Review*, 87, 102038. https://doi.org/10.1016/j.cpr.2021.102038

47 Twenge, J. M., Joiner, T. E., Rogers, M. L., & Martin, G. N. (2018). Increases in depressive symptoms, suicide-related outcomes, and suicide rates among U.S. adolescents after 2010 and links to increased new-media screen time. *Clinical Psychological Science*, 6(1), 3–17. https://doi.org/10.1177/2167702617723376

48 Marchant, A., Hawton, K., Stewart, A., Montgomery, P., Singaravelu, V., Lloyd, K., Purdy, N., Daine, K., & John, A. (2017). A systematic review of the relationship between internet use, self-harm and suicidal behaviour in young people: The good, the bad and the unknown. PLOS ONE, 12(8), e0181722. https://doi.org/10.1371/journal.pone.0181722

49 Office of the Surgeon General. (2023). Social media and youth mental health: The U.S. Surgeon General's advisory. U.S. Department of Health and Human Services. https://www.hhs.gov/surgeongeneral/reports-and-publications/youth-mental-health/index.html

50 Robinson, J., Hill, N. T. M., Thorn, P., Teh, Z., & Lamblin, M. (2024). Social media and suicide risk in youth: A review. JAMA Network Open, 7(5), e2412579. https://doi.org/10.1001/jamanetworkopen.2024.12579

51 Exploding Topics. (2025, July 23). Worldwide daily social media usage (new 2025 data). Retrieved from [https://explodingtopics.com/blog/social-media-usage?utm_source=chatgpt.com#daily-time-social-media]

52 Coccaro, E. F., Lee, R., & McCloskey, M. S. (2015). Serotonin and impulsive aggression. *Central Nervous System Agents in Medicinal Chemistry*, 15(4), 289–297. https://doi.org/10.2174/1871524915666150716104929

53 Berridge, K. C., & Kringelbach, M. L. (2015). Pleasure systems in the brain. *Neuron*, 86(3), 646–664. https://doi.org/10.1016/j.neuron.2015.02.018

54 Corsi-Cabrera, M., Velasco, F., Del Río-Portilla, Y., Armony, J. L.,

Trejo-Martínez, D., Guevara, M. A., & Velasco, A. L. (2016). Human amygdala activation during rapid eye movements of rapid eye movement sleep: an intracranial study. *Journal of sleep research*, 25(5), 576–582. https://doi.org/10.1111/jsr.12415

55 Stothard, E.R., McHill, A. W., Depner, C.M., Birks, B. R., Moehlman, T. M., Ritchie, H. K., ...Wright, K. P. (2017). "Circadian entrainment to the natural light-dark cycle across seasons and the weekend," *Current Biology*, 27(4), 508-513.

56 Ibid.

57 Congressional Budget Office. (2021, April). Research and development in the pharmaceutical industry (Report No. 57126). https://www.cbo.gov/publication/57126

58 Krystal, A. D., Walsh, J. K., Laska, E., Caron, J., Amato, D. A., Wessel, T., & Roth, T. (2003). Sustained efficacy of eszopiclone over 6 months of nightly treatment: Results of a randomized, double-blind, placebo-controlled study in adults with chronic insomnia. *Sleep*, 26(7), 793–799. https://doi.org/10.1093/sleep/26.7.793

59 Burns, A. C., Saxena, R., Vetter, C., Phillips, A. J. K., Lane, J. M., & Cain, S. W. (2021). "Time spent in outdoor light is associated with mood, sleep, and circadian rhythm-related outcomes: A cross-sectional and longitudinal study in over 400,000 UK Biobank participants," *Journal of affective disorders*, 295, 347–352. https://doi.org/10.1016/j.jad.2021.08.056

60 These articles comprise the most foundational ideas for the Camping In Reset.

Eto, T., Kitamura, S., Nishimura, K., Takeoka, K., Nishimura, Y., Lee, S. I.,... & Higuchi, S. (2022). "Circadian phase advances in children during camping life according to the natural light-dark cycle," *Journal of physiological anthropology*, *41*(1), 42.

Stothard, E.R., McHill, A. W., Depner, C.M., Birks, B. R., Moehlman, T. M., Ritchie, H. K., ...Wright, K. P. (2017). "Circadian entrainment to the natural light-dark cycle across seasons and the weekend," *Current Biology, 27(4), 508-513.*

Burns, A. C., Saxena, R., Vetter, C., Phillips, A. J. K., Lane, J. M., & Cain, S. W. (2021). "Time spent in outdoor light is associated with mood, sleep, and circadian rhythm-related outcomes: A cross-sectional and longitudinal study in over 400,000 UK Biobank participants," *Journal of affective disorders*, *295*, 347–352. https://doi.org/10.1016/j.jad.2021.08.056

61 Vandewalle, G., Middleton, B., Senechal, M., Lê Minh, N., Dumont, M., Vandewalle, N., Delius, J. D., Gabel, V., Vu, T. C., & Carrier, J. (2006). Repeated exposures to daytime bright light increase nocturnal

melatonin rise and maintain circadian phase in young subjects under fixed sleep schedule. *American Journal of Physiology - Regulatory, Integrative and Comparative Physiology*, 290(5), R1233-R1240. https://doi.org/10.1152/ajpregu.00211.2006

62 Bano-Otalora, B., Martial, F., Harding, C., Bechtold, D. A., Allen, A. E., Brown, T. M., Belle, M. D. C., & Lucas, R. J. (2021). Bright daytime light enhances circadian amplitude in a diurnal mammal. Proceedings of the National Academy of Sciences of the United States of America, 118(22), e2100094118. https://doi.org/10.1073/pnas.2100094118

63 Frontiers in Nutrition. (2020). Feeding Rhythms and the Circadian Regulation of Metabolism. *Frontiers in Nutrition*, 7, Article 39. https://doi.org/10.3389/fnut.2020.00039

64 Gill, S., & Panda, S. (2015). A smartphone app reveals erratic diurnal eating patterns in humans that can be modulated for health benefits. *Cell Metabolism*, 22(5), 789–798. https://doi.org/10.1016/j.cmet.2015.09.005

65 Tahara, Y., & Shibata, S. (2013). Chronobiology and nutrition. *Journal of Biological Rhythms*, 28(4), 283–289. https://doi.org/10.1177/0748730413493862

66 Czerwony, B. (2024, December 9). How to get caffeine out of your system. Cleveland Clinic. https://health.clevelandclinic.org/how-to-get-caffeine-out-of-your-system/

# ACKNOWLEDGMENTS

My friend Justin is a fantastic author. He told me once that he became a writer because it was the only thing teachers never told him to stop doing. For me, that has been sleep work—no one ever told me to stop doing it. Along the way, I was encouraged and shown the next level by several mentors. I owe them everything.

I mentioned Dr. Song Ping Lee as the ear, nose, throat doctor who first diagnosed my deviated septum and then surgically fixed it. I owe him my professional career, at least, but also my health and possibly my life.

Once I could sleep well, I realized how important sleep was and immediately signed up for one of the few courses on sleep and dreaming in the country in 1989, taught by Dr. Charles Hallenbeck at the University of Kansas. Dr. Hallenbeck's academic starting place gave me an awareness of a larger scientific community and encouraged me to continue looking for new developments, which I continue to do. I am disappointed that it is too late to tell Song Ping and Charles how much I appreciate them before their deaths.

Dr. Kathy Miller was a professor at Temple University and my first mentor who saw the passion I had for sleep and worked with me on my first publication. She saw the possibilities and helped me believe that I had something to say that people could use.

Professionally, I have so many people to thank for encouraging me and showing me how I could develop in this field. Dr. Jodi Mindell at St. Joseph's University and the Children's Hospital of Philadelphia, the brilliant pediatric sleep psychologist I bumped into in 1998, is one of the kindest, most empathic, and encouraging people. She treated me as a colleague right away, despite how little I knew or understood about what I was doing.

Without Dr. Phil German at the University of Pennsylvania, I wouldn't have been able to treat the hundreds (thousands?) of clients I have seen over the years. Phil took his own time and supervised me outside of his busy work schedule and family life because he wanted to help me. Phil's generosity and supervision made it possible for me to become board certified.

Dr. Charles Beale at the University of Delaware was my boss to whom I owe similar gratitude for allowing me to get the training and supervision I needed alongside my work duties. He didn't have to, but he wanted to encourage me to develop my professional passion. As I got to know him better, I came to understand that this is what he does best—he's a genius at helping people develop their passions.

Since then, I have had so much encouragement and help from audiences I've talked to about sleep, from my clients, my kids Henry and Claire, my friends, and the rest of my family to put together my thoughts in book form. While my kids were probably the first to suggest I write a book—they may have been trying to find a way to get me to tell someone *else* about sleep for a change, lol.

Myles Schrag, a friend from another time and place, came back into my life at the right time. I don't rely on luck to show me my path, but I try not to miss the obvious moments when the universe reintroduces a trusted old friend who happens to work with authors like me. Myles has been kind, patient, passionate, and professional. Myles introduced me to Sarah Herse, an editor with a kind heart and a keen eye for clarity, consistency, and citations.

Early readers of this book who provided me with direction and encouragement include the intrepid Daniel Kim, LCSW, DBSM, and the amazing Virginia Runko, PhD, CBSM, DBSM. These two are amazing human beings and amazing sleep clinicians at the top of their professional games. This book would have been far worse without them.

Another early reader was Larry Wolgast, my dad. Not a sleep expert, but a voracious reader and someone easy for me to trust. The direction and suggestions he gave were exceptionally helpful. He and my mom have always supported me through all my decisions. I can never repay the love, kindness, warmth, and support I have received being their son.

Most of all, my wife and bed-partner, Lisa. Lisa has been my number one supporter and encourager, going through ideas, good and bad, for what should be included as well as the highs and lows that come from living with me through a journey into doing something neither of us has ever done before. I couldn't ask for a better partner in all things.

# ABOUT THE AUTHOR

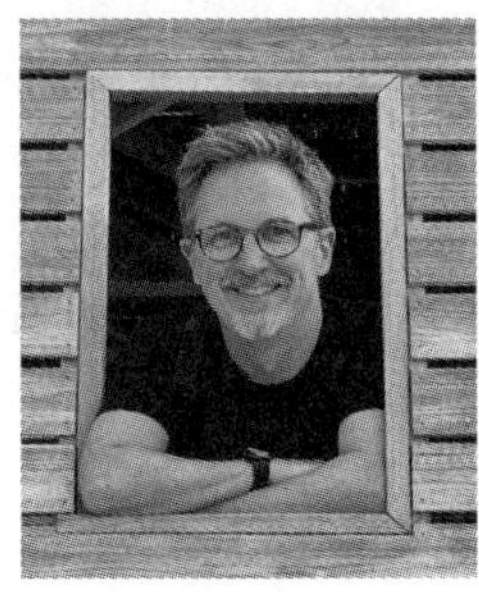

Brad Wolgast, PhD, DBSM, is a licensed psychologist and board certified in behavioral sleep medicine. He suffered from a sleep disorder his entire childhood. Getting healthy sleep changed his life, so for more than two decades his passion has been the study of sleep and helping a wide range of people to experience better sleep.

Dr. Wolgast worked at the University of Pennsylvania and the University of Delaware and now operates the Center for Healthy Sleep, LLC. He works extensively with athletes and university teams to improve their sleep and performance, as well as treating people suffering from insomnia and chronic nightmares. Dr. Wolgast speaks nationally to health care providers and groups about how to use human mechanisms for superior sleep and overall health.

In his free time, Brad is a slow runner and an even slower cyclist. He lives in Southeastern Pennsylvania with his wife, though they leave often to seek out the mountains.

centerforhealthysleep